Interpreting
Dental Radiographs

Interpreting Dental Radiographs

Brian W. Beeching

M.PHIL, M.SC, BDS, LDSRCS

Senior Demonstrator in charge of the
Dental Radiology Department,
Guy's Hospital Dental School,
London

1981

UPDATE BOOKS

LONDON/DORDRECHT/BOSTON

Available in the United Kingdom and Eire
from

Update Books Ltd
33-34 Alfred Place
London WC1E 7DP
England

Available in the USA and Canada from

Kluwer Boston Inc.
Lincoln Building, 190 Old Derby Street
Hingham, Mass. 02043
USA

Available in the rest of the World from

Kluwer Academic Publishers
Group Distribution Centre
PO Box 322, 3300 AH Dordrecht
The Netherlands

First Published 1981

© *Update Books Ltd 1981*

British Library Cataloguing in Publication Data

Beeching, Brian
Interpreting dental radiographs.
1. Teeth—Radiography
I. Title
617.6'07'57   RK309

ISBN 0-906141-20-6

ISBN 0 906141 20 6
Production by R. James Hall
Book Production Services
Text set in Times Roman, 10pt on 12pt, with Univers
Printed in Great Britain by
Cradley Printing Co. Ltd,
Cradley Heath, West Midlands

Contents

Acknowledgements

Acknowledgements are due to past and present consultants, members of staff and students of Guy's Dental Hospital and School whose patients have indirectly provided the radiographic illustrations.

I am indebted to: Mrs E. Jaffe, Dept of Dentistry for Children for Figures 268, 269, 270 and 271; Mr P. Longhurst, Dept of Dentistry for Children for Figure 267; Mr L. Usiskin, Dept of Orthodontics for Figure 243; Mr J. Radford, Dept of Preventive Dentistry for Figure 264; and Ms A. Wyatt, Newcastle Dental School Hospital (and the Graves Medical Audiovisual Library) for Plates 1, 2 & 3.

I am indebted to Dr W. Campbell, Consultant Radiologist at Queen Victoria Hospital, East Grinstead, who has kindly provided examples of the Le Fort fractures from his collection.

Particular acknowledgements and thanks are due to Dr Frank Ingram, Consultant Dental Radiologist at Guy's for many years, who stimulated my interest in the speciality. Since his retirement in 1978 Dr Ingram's carefully stored hoard of radiographs has been plundered unmercilessly to provide many of the illustrations to go with this text.

Throughout this book I have searched diligently for the sources of all the radiographs used. I acknowledge that this has not always been possible and offer apologies for the very few for which I may have failed to give due credit.

Thanks are due to the staff of Update Books, in particular Maggie Pettifer for her interest and enthusiasm, Karen Williams for her meticulous editing, and Howard Prescott for his patience in producing all the art work.

Finally, I would like to thank my wife Ruth for her constant consideration and understanding, without which this book would not have been possible.

Preface

The title *Interpreting Dental Radiographs* indicates the intended practical nature of this book.

It is hoped that students, practitioners, dental radiologists and senior radiographers will find this straightforward volume a useful chairside companion, as it covers the common, and some of the more rare, radiological appearances seen within the field of dentistry.

Medical radiologists should find the text and related radiographic examples a useful supplement to their knowledge of general radiology.

The writer has attempted to indicate that interpretation of dental radiographs is not always simple and straightforward, particularly when considering periapical changes and neoplasms. Careful assessment of the whole radiograph is essential to avoid the pitfall of developing 'tunnel vision'!

No apology is given for the repetitive indication of the types of radiographic views necessary to illustrate structures and pathological processes. It is hoped that this will make students realise the importance of requesting the correct radiographic views for the condition under consideration.

The few references given should open the field of further reading to those interested in dental radiology.

Brian W. Beeching
Guy's Hospital, London
December 1980

1. Normal Anatomy

Both the general practitioner and the consultant radiologist have to differentiate between the pathological and the wide variations of the normal when assessing radiographs. Their assessment is based only on differing degrees of radiolucency and opacity on what is, to all intents and purposes, a shadowgraph.

Detail is of the utmost importance in interpretation as dental structures are usually small, and early assessment of caries, and pulpal and bone changes is essential.

It is for this reason that non-screen film is still used in dentistry, and that the film is made in sizes suitable for insertion into the mouth, so that it can be positioned as closely as possible to the area under investigation.

When the dental surgeon requires information on the extent of fractures, the size of lesions, the presence or absence of teeth and the size and shape of jaws, he will use screen film in cassettes. The exposure time is greatly reduced compared with non-screen film, but at the same time detail is lost.

The Tooth and Supporting Structure

The tissues making up the tooth and its supporting structure can be well illustrated on the bitewing radiograph (Figure 1).

The enamel presents as a dense radio-opaque band covering the crown of the tooth and ending as a tapering edge at the neck of the tooth. Breaks in the smooth outline, both on the outside and at the amelodentinal junction are evident when caries or trauma has occurred.

The dentine lies immediately below the enamel and comprises the bulk of the crown and the whole of the root. Dentine is less opaque than enamel, but of similar density to compact bone. The caries process can be seen as a radiolucency of the dentine.

The pulp, being soft tissue, is a continuous radiolucent chamber extending from the crown of the tooth to the apex of the root. The size and shape of this radiolucent chamber are all important in the assessment of its condition.

The cementum covers the root of the tooth as a very thin layer, and is not discernible on radiographs unless hypercementosis has occurred. The bulbous nature of the root is then obvious (Figure 128) and the opacity is usually similar to that of dentine though it is sometimes more radiolucent.

The periodontal membrane is depicted as a very narrow radiolucent line immediately surrounding the root of the tooth. The condition of this supporting

Figure 1. *Right bitewing radiograph showing the relative densities of enamel, dentine, pulp, periodontal membrane, bone and amalgam filling material.*

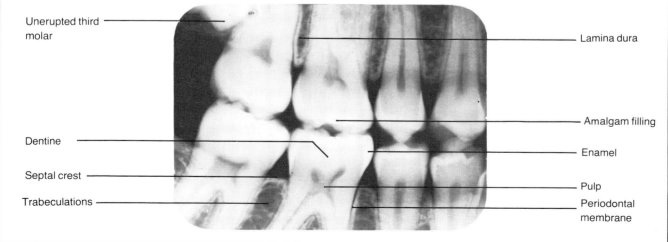

Unerupted third molar

Dentine

Septal crest

Trabeculations

Lamina dura

Amalgam filling

Enamel

Pulp

Periodontal membrane

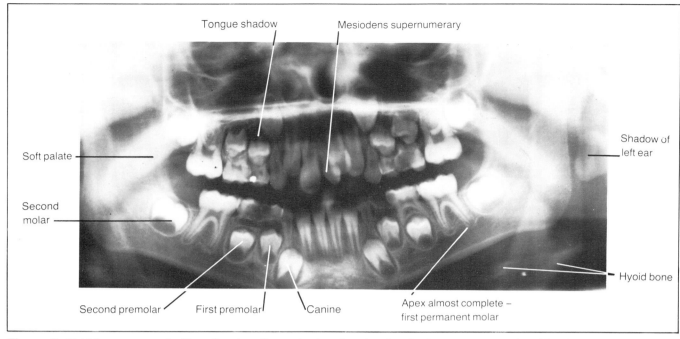

Tongue shadow

Mesiodens supernumerary

Soft palate

Second molar

Shadow of left ear

Second premolar

First premolar

Canine

Apex almost complete – first permanent molar

Hyoid bone

Figure 2. *Orbiting panoramic (Panelipse) radiograph showing the developing permanent dentition in an eight-year-old child.*

structure is assessed by noting the even width throughout its extent, and the condition of the harder structures that border it, the cementum/dentine and lamina dura.

The lamina dura, the dense compact bone of the tooth socket, is an even radio-opaque line surrounding the root of the tooth and continuous across the interdental crest in the healthy subject. Absence at any point of the lamina is highly indicative of infection, trauma or underlying disease processes. Therefore it is one of the most important landmarks on a radiograph.

The Developing Tooth

The Panelipse (orbiting panoramic) radiograph (Figure 2) shows the developing permanent dentition in a child aged eight years. The very carious deciduous molars are also shown.

Crypts of the third molars are not yet evident, but should be seen by 10 years of age. Crowns of $\frac{7543 \mid 3457}{7543 \mid 3457}$ are complete, and root formation has commenced in the canines.

Figure 3. *Panelipse radiograph showing developing third molars in a child aged 12 years. The coronoid process of the mandible and the shadow of the soft palate frequently obscure the crypts of the developing upper third molars.*

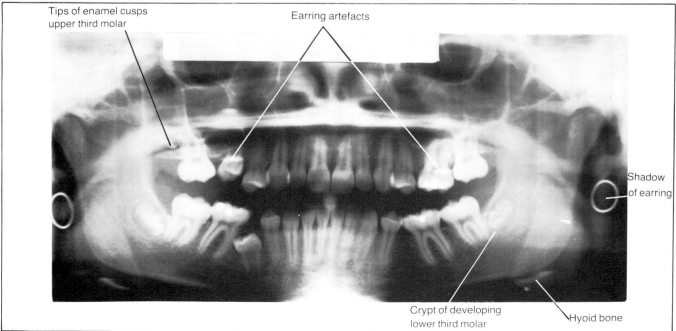

Tips of enamel cusps upper third molar

Earring artefacts

Shadow of earring

Crypt of developing lower third molar

Hyoid bone

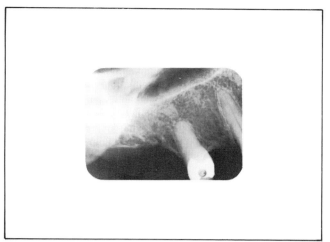

Figure 4. *Periapical radiograph 65| region showing normal trabecular bone pattern in the maxilla.*

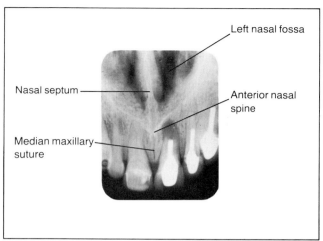

Figure 6. *Periapical radiograph 1|1 region showing the nasal fossa, nasal septum and the anterior nasal spine.*

The apices of the lower first molars are not quite complete and care has to be taken not to confuse the remaining radicular papilla with a developing area of bone change following death of the pulp. There is a mesiodens preventing eruption of |1 into the arch.

The Panelipse view (Figure 3), shows developing third molars in a girl aged 12 years. The opacity of the soft palate and coronoid process of the mandible frequently obscures the developing upper third molar region, making early assessment of these teeth difficult on this type of radiograph.

Earrings project the shadows seen in 5|6 regions.

The Maxilla

The maxilla is a more fibrous bone than the mandible and as a result its trabeculations are less dense and coarse than the latter's. The trabeculations are depicted on the radiograph as fine lace-like opacities (Figure 4).

The median suture of the maxilla can sometimes, though by no means always, be seen on radiographs of younger patients (Figure 5). It presents as a radiolucent line running from the incisal crest of bone between the two upper central incisors.

The nasal fossa (Figure 6) is outlined on the periapical view of the upper incisor region by opaque lines, which are themselves bisected by the *nasal septum,* all joining together to form the opacity of the *anterior nasal spine.*

Closely related to the nasal spine is the *anterior palatine fossa,* an oval or round radiolucency between, above or superimposed on the apices of the upper central incisors on radiographic views of these teeth. As anterior palatine foramina can vary considerably in size (Figure 7), it makes assessment as to when a cyst of the anterior palatine canal is present difficult.

It is most important for us to be able to differentiate between the anterior palatine fossa and an area of bone change at the apex of a central incisor. Further con-

Figure 5. *Periapical view 1|1 region showing median suture of the maxilla.*

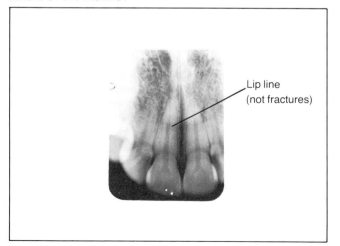

Figure 7. *Periapical radiograph 1|1 region showing anterior palatine fossa.*

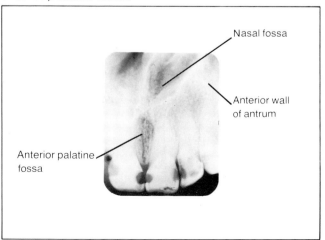

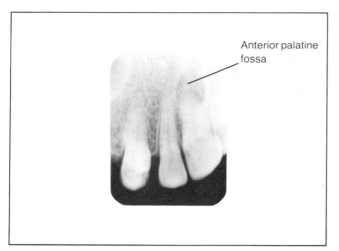

Figure 8. *Periapical view 2⌋ showing anterior palatine fossa projected over the apex 1⌋.*

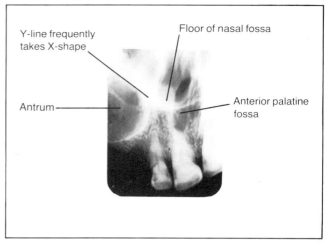

Figure 10. *Periapical radiograph 2⌋ region illustrating the 'X'-line. This occurs when the anterior wall of the antrum crosses over the nasal floor and continues upwards.*

fusion is added because the foramen or fossa's shadow will fall directly over a central incisor when centring is through the adjacent lateral incisor (Figure 8).

Periapical radiographs of the upper canine region will frequently demonstrate a landmark termed the *Y-line of Ennis*.

Opaque lines, the floor of the nasal fossa and the anterior boundary of the maxillary antrum, join to form an inverted 'Y' (Figure 9). On occasions the 'Y' becomes an 'X', when the opaque line of the anterior wall of the antrum crosses the floor of the nasal fossa and continues as a separate opaque line (Figure 10).

The maxillary antrum can vary enormously in size and shape, and is readily evident in all radiographs of

upper premolar and molar regions (Figures 11 and 12). Generally it commences behind the upper canine as a radiolucent area and extends backwards towards the maxillary tuberosity. Sometimes it extends further forwards (Figure 13) to the lateral incisor region.

The antral floor may be well above the roots of the premolar and molar teeth, or it may dip down between the roots reaching almost to the alveolar crest, the roots appearing as finger-like processes poking up into the antrum, though still covered by lamina dura.

Compartments or loculations are frequently evident, and differential diagnosis with cyst has to be made with care, the lamina dura playing an important part in this assessment. Sometimes the left and right antra will be

Figure 9. *Periapical radiograph ⌊34 region illustrating the inverted 'Y'-line of Ennis. The anterior wall of the antrum rises to join the floor of the nose.*

Figure 11. *Periapical radiograph 54⌋ region showing large antrum.*

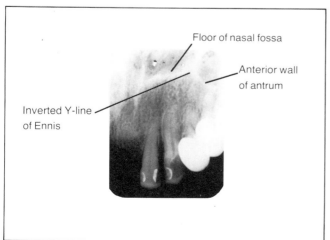

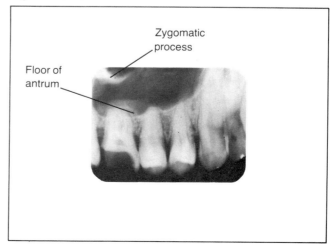

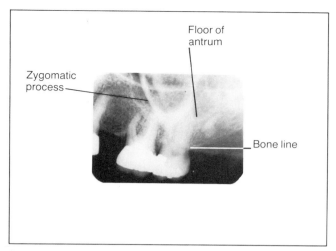

Figure 12. *Periapical radiograph* $\underline{\,7}$ *region showing normal antrum above molars.*

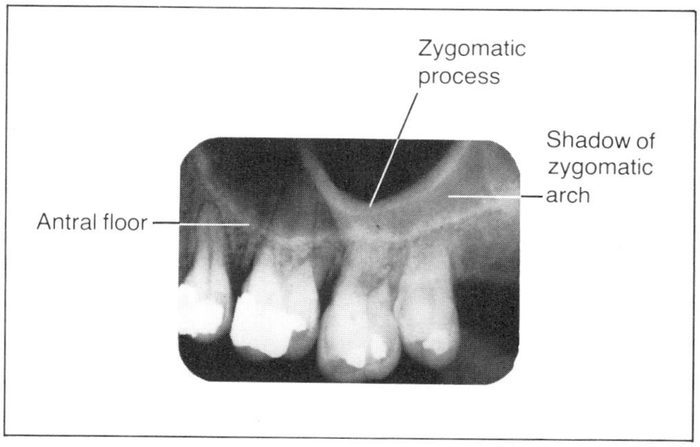

Figure 14. *Bisected angle technique radiographs showing the U-shaped shadow of the zygomatic buttress falling over the upper molar roots.*

quite different in size and shape, adding to the confusion of interpretation!

Vascular grooves can sometimes be seen as radiolucent channels running across the walls of the antrum and these help in the differential diagnosis between antrum and cyst.

The antral cavity often extends out into the *zygomatic process*. The zygomatic buttress casts a 'V'- or 'U'-shaped opacity on to the radiograph in most cases over the roots of the first and second molars (Figure 14), particularly where the bisected angle technique has been used (Figure 15).

A long cone paralleling technique radiograph of the upper molar region (Figure 16) will remove the zygo-

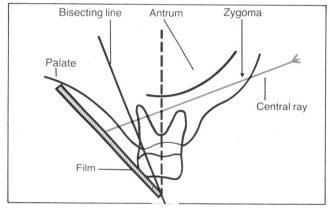

Figure 15. *Diagram illustrating the bisected angle technique in* $\underline{\,6}$ *region. This shows why the shadow of the zygomatic buttress falls over the roots of the upper molars on this type of radiograph.*

Figure 13. *Periapical radiograph* $\underline{21}$ *region showing large antrum extending forwards to* $\underline{2\,}$ *region.*

Figure 16. *Paralleling technique radiograph* $\underline{\,6}$*region showing shadow of zygoma away from the apices of the upper molars, making interpretation of this area possible.*

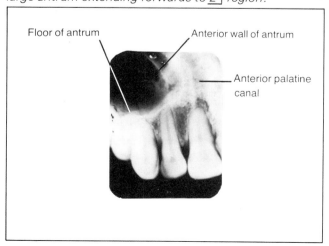

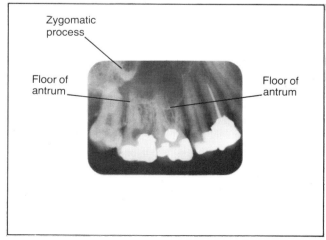

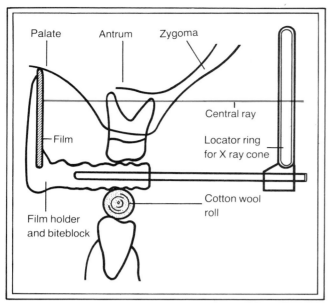

Figure 17. *Diagram of the paralleling technique, showing the horizontal central ray passing below the zygomatic process. The zygoma's shadow will then be projected higher on the radiograph and away from the apices of the upper molars.*

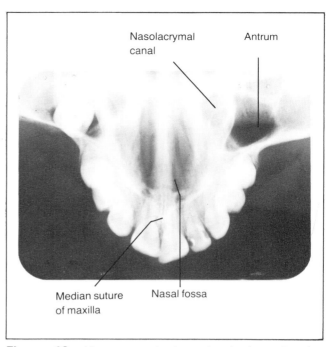

Figure 19. *Upper standard occlusal view showing nasolacrymal canals, antra, nasal fossae and median suture of the maxilla.*

matic shadow from over the apices of the teeth. This technique (Figure 17) is advised routinely for all periapical views of the upper molars.

Because the film cannot be brought close to the teeth being radiographed there will be magnification of the image unless a long cone is used on the x-ray set (Updegrave 1971).

The zygomatic arch, when evident, is a wide radio-opaque band extending posteriorly from the zygomatic process (Figure 14).

The outline of the *maxillary tuberosity* can be seen in radiographs of the upper third molar region, and sometimes the shadow of the *coronoid process* of the mandible can be seen in this region when the jaws are in close proximity (Figure 18).

Occasionally the *pterygoid hamulus* with its characteristic outline will stand out as a radio-opacity posteriorly to the tuberosity (Figure 18).

The *nasolacrymal canals* can often be seen on the standard occlusal radiograph, and because of the angle of projection are seen as oval or round radiolucent areas posteriorly on the hard palate (Figure 19) (Smith 1980).

Figure 18. *Periapical radiograph 87\ region showing zygomatic arch shadow, tuberosity, pterygoid hamulus and coronoid process of the mandible.*

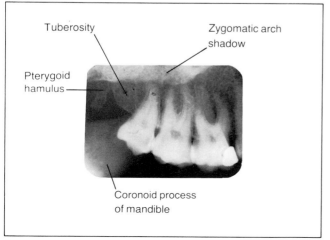

Figure 20. *Periapical radiograph ⌐678 region showing the trabecular pattern of mandibular bone and cortex of the lower border.*

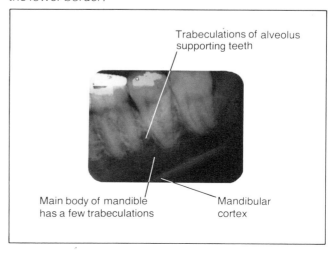

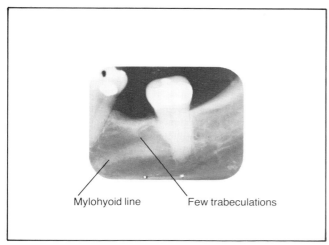

Mylohyoid line   Few trabeculations

Figure 21. *Periapical radiograph* $\overline{8}$ *region showing mandible with sparse trabeculations.*

Inferior dental canal

Dense trabeculations

Figure 22. *Periapical radiograph* $\overline{8}$ *region showing mandible with dense trabeculations.*

The Mandible

The trabecular bone of the mandible is generally more dense and coarse than that of the maxilla. The cortex is thicker and casts a very dense shadow (Figure 20).

The trabeculae are mainly aligned horizontally and can vary considerably in quantity from patient to patient (Figures 21 and 22).

The condylar head can be seen in the Panelipse radiograph (Figure 23), as can the other basic components of the mandible: the *coronoid process, ramus, angle, body* and *symphysis.*

Figure 23 also shows the course of the *inferior dental canal* from its opening below the sigmoid notch at the lingula towards the mental region. This radiolucent

Figure 23. *Panelipse radiograph of man of 53 years showing main components of mandible: coronoid process, condyle, ramus, angle, body, symphysis and the inferior dental canal. The patient's left side of the mandible has been outlined to aid the identification of the structures.*

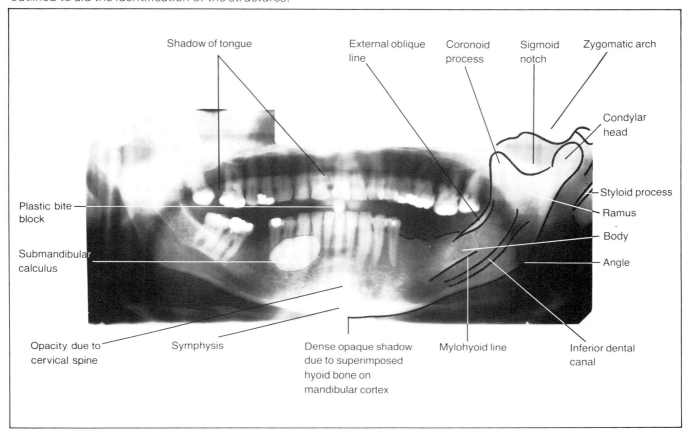

Shadow of tongue

External oblique line

Coronoid process

Sigmoid notch

Zygomatic arch

Condylar head

Plastic bite block

Submandibular calculus

Styloid process

Ramus

Body

Angle

Opacity due to cervical spine

Symphysis

Dense opaque shadow due to superimposed hyoid bone on mandibular cortex

Mylohyoid line

Inferior dental canal

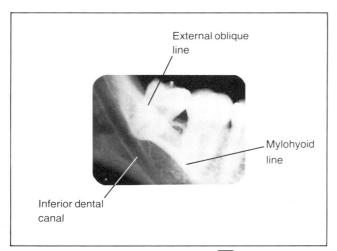

Figure 24. *Periapical radiograph* $\overline{8|}$ *region. Heavy opaque band at the apices* $\overline{86|}$ *($\overline{7|}$ is missing) is the mylohyoid line. Below this the radiolucent area with fewer trabeculations houses the inferior dental canal with lightly opaque upper and lower borders. The external oblique ridge presents as an opaque band across the neck of* $\overline{8|}$ *.*

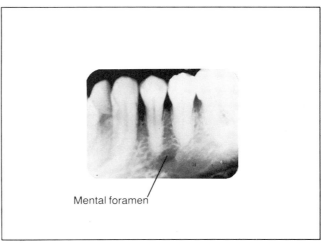

Figure 26. *Periapical radiograph* $\overline{|3\text{-}6}$ *region. The mental foramen can be seen as an oval radiolucency between the roots of* $\overline{|45}$ *. Confusion can be made with an apical area when this dark area falls over the apices of either permanent premolar. An intact lamina dura settles the diagnosis as mental foramen.*

canal is generally outlined by opaque lines and shows up well on periapical radiographs of the third molar region. On occasions the canal will present as a radiolucent or opaque band, or it may be invisible on the radiograph altogether (Figure 24).

The canal is important as a radiographic landmark,

Figure 25. *Periapical radiograph* $\overline{6\text{-}3|}$ *region. The inferior dental canal and mental foramen can all be seen on this radiograph. The mental canal can be seen to run upwards and backwards from its junction with the inferior dental canal.*

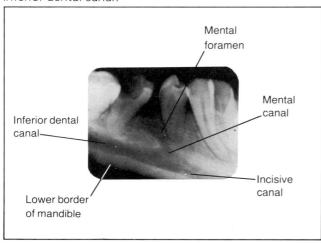

close proximity with the roots of the lower third molar being all important when removal of the latter is indicated.

The external oblique ridge of the mandible (Figure 24) usually presents as a radio-opaque band crossing the neck of the lower third molar from its origin on the ramus to its insertion in the body of the mandible.

The mylohyoid line (Figure 24), on the lingual aspect of the mandible, is generally evident as a narrow opaque band crossing the roots or below the apices of the lower first, second and third molars. Very often the trabeculations below this line will be less dense and less frequent than in the alveolar tooth-supporting part above.

Differentiation has to be made between the external oblique line, the mylohyoid line and the inferior dental canal when assessing radiographs of the lower second and third molar regions.

The mental foramen appears as an oval or round radiolucency within the immediate neighbourhood of the apices of the permanent premolars (Figures 25 and 26). The foramen may appear to be superimposed over the apex of either premolar, and has to be differentiated from an area of periapical infection.

The tributary *mental canal* leading to the mental foramen can sometimes be traced from its junction with the inferior dental canal (Figure 25), as can the continuation of the latter, the *incisive canal*.

Occasionally an incisive foramen or genial pit can be seen in the midline of the mandible below the apices of the incisors (Figure 27). It is usually positioned between the genial tubercles, or slightly above them, and is easily found on the dried skull. It may conduct anastomosing vessels.

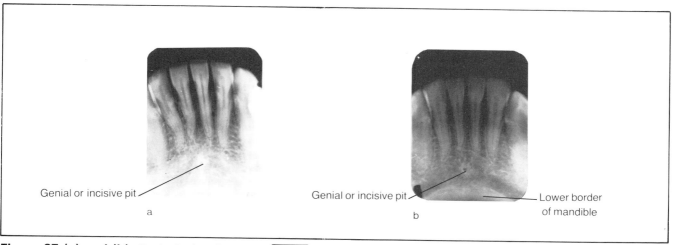

Genial or incisive pit

a

Genial or incisive pit Lower border of mandible

b

Figure 27 (a) and (b). *Periapical radiographs* $\overline{21\,|\,12}$ *regions to show genial or incisive pit/foramen, usually found between or above the genial tubercles on the lingual surface of the mandible.*

The mental eminences often present as dense opaque bands below the apices of the lower anterior teeth meeting in the midline (Figure 28).

The genial tubercles stand out as triangular opacities of varying sizes on the true lower occlusal radiographic view (Figure 29).

Figure 30 illustrates *nutrient vessels* running vertically in the mandible as radiolucent channels. They are not easy to see in reproductions of radiographs. In dentate jaws these channels can be seen to reach up into the interdental and inter-radicular crest bone, as well as terminating at the apical regions of the teeth.

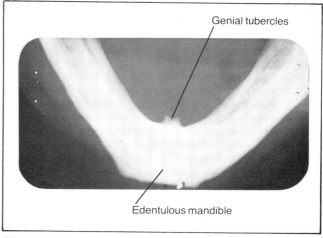

Genial tubercles

Edentulous mandible

Figure 29. *True lower occlusal view of edentulous mandible showing opaque genial tubercles. These can vary considerably in size and shape.*

Figure 30. *Periapical radiograph showing vertical nutrient vessels in the anterior region of a dentate mandible. These can, on occasions, also be seen in views of the maxilla.*

Figure 28. *Periapical radiograph* $\overline{21\,|\,12}$ *region to show the mental eminences.*

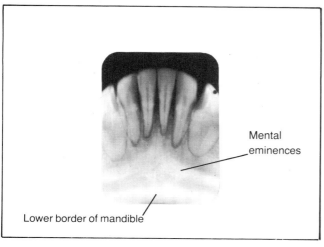

Mental eminences

Lower border of mandible

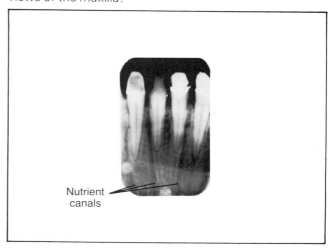

Nutrient canals

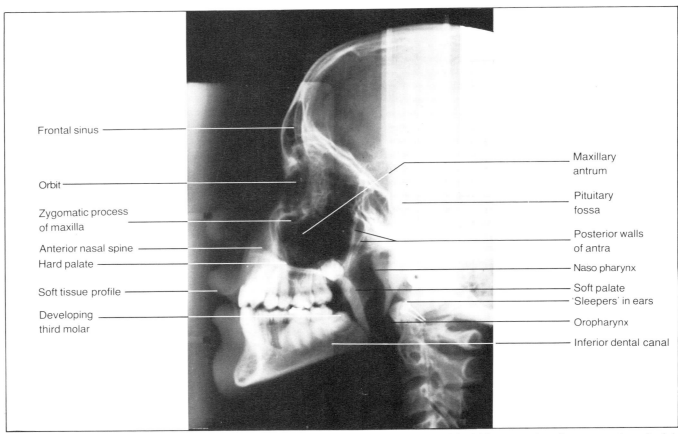

Figure 31. *True lateral skull radiograph, with the patient in a craniostat, of a girl of 12 years showing general orofacial anatomy.*

Figure 32. *Panelipse radiograph illustrating anatomy of the orofacial region. One side of the mandible has been outlined to aid in identification of the structures.*

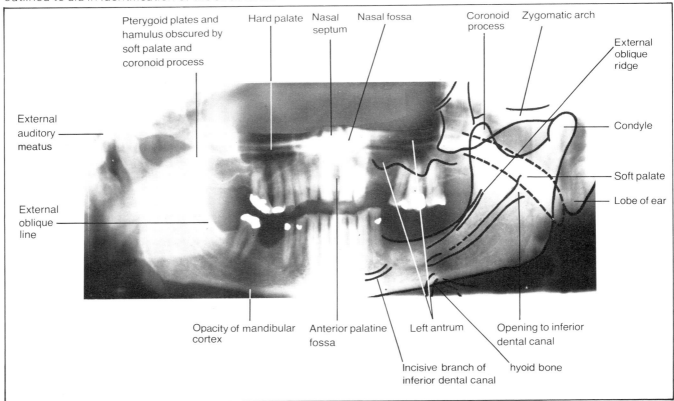

General Orofacial Anatomy

Figure 31, a true lateral skull view in the craniostat, and Figure 32, a Panelipse view, illustrate radiographically the normal anatomy of the orofacial region, and demonstrate the structures of interest to the dental surgeon.

It has to be borne in mind with all extraoral radiographs that superimposed shadows will be cast by overlying structures, leading on occasions to a difficulty in diagnosis. The air shadows can be troublesome and confusing in this respect, as can the hyoid bone, particularly so on an oblique lateral view.

References

Smith, N. J. D., *Dental Radiography*, Blackwell Scientific Publications, Oxford, 1980 p.74.

Updegrave, W. J., *New Horizons in Periapical and Interproximal Radiography*, Rinn Corporation, Elgin, Illinois, 1971.

2. Developmental Abnormalities

Orofacial Abnormalities

There are a considerable number of possible orofacial abnormalities, some related to specific syndromes and others chance occurrences. Two examples only are considered, both demonstrating the considerable variations that can occur in growth of the mandible.

Mandibular Prognathism

Figure 33, a true lateral skull projection with the patient in a craniostat, illustrates mandibular prognathism with overgrowth of the mandible. The original radiograph shows the facial contour associated with this condition. Soft tissue profiles can be produced on radiographs by placing an aluminium wedge between the x-ray beam and the patient at the point of interest, in this case the nose, lips and chin. The wedge stops sufficient of the radiation to enable the facial contour to be seen. A true lateral radiographic projection showing the soft tissue profile is of considerable assistance to the oral surgeon who is proposing to correct the condition.

Underdevelopment of the Mandible

Figure 34 demonstrates the condition of 'bird-face' and under-development of the mandible. Again, a true lateral projection with soft tissue profile is a help to the oral surgeon.

The examples shown are extremes, and there are many cases that fall part-way between the two.

Unilateral Micro- and Macrognathia

Unilateral micro- and macrognathia can occur, resulting in a lop-sided appearance. A submentovertex radiograph is taken in these cases which shows any lateral deviation of the jaws. Figure 35 illustrates the position of the patient for this view of the skull.

Figure 33. *True lateral skull in a craniostat, showing mandibular prognathism. The facial contour has been marked in for clarification though it can easily be seen on the original radiograph.*

Figure 34. *True lateral skull in craniostat showing 'bird-face' and underdevelopment of the mandible. The facial contour has been marked in for clarification.*

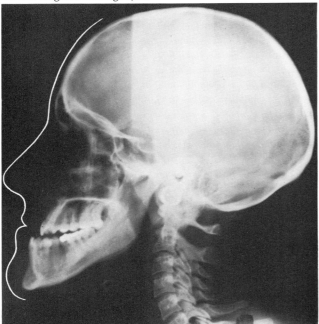

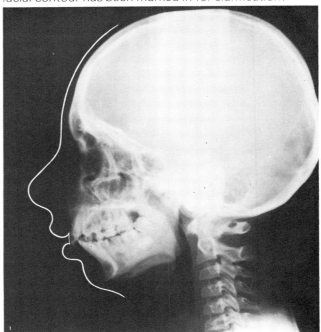

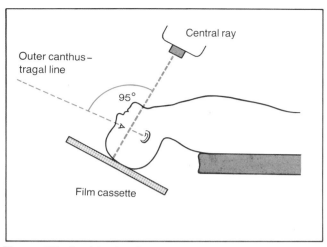

Figure 35. *Positioning for submentovertex radiographic view of the skull.*

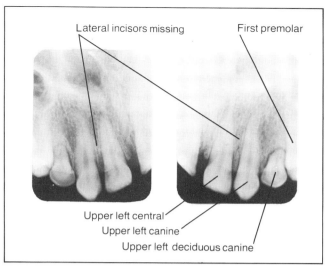

Figure 37. *Periapical radiographs of the upper anteriors demonstrating absence of lateral incisors, 3|3 taking up the laterals' position, and C|C retained in 3|3 position.*

Tooth Abnormalities

Missing Teeth

The condition of congenitally missing teeth is quite common and may follow a hereditary pattern. Any tooth in the dental arch may be absent, but the most common absentee is the third molar, followed by the second premolar (Figure 36), and the upper lateral incisor (Figure 37). Missing teeth may be unilateral, bilateral or from all four quadrants.

The term oligodontia is reserved for those cases where there are multiples of teeth missing, and this occurs in ectodermal dysplasia, a syndrome characterized by complete or partial absence of the sweat glands. The

hair follicles are often defective or absent. Anodontia may occur in these individuals, though it is more usual for a few teeth to be present (Figure 38).

It has been known for teeth to be missing in children following x-ray therapy to the developing jaws in the treatment of neoplasia. This is probably due to the fact that the developing tooth buds are very sensitive to x-radiation (Shafer et al. 1958).

Macro- and Microdontia

Macrodontia may affect the complete dentition, in which case it is probably the result of hyperpituitarism.

Figure 36. *Oblique lateral view of the right mandible showing retention of E| and absence of 5|. The cervical spine obscures 8|, so assessment of development of the lower third molar is not possible.*

Figure 38. *Periapical radiographs of lower jaw of a 19-year-old girl with oligodontia. 6| unfortunately had to be removed due to caries, leaving only E4C|C6 standing.*

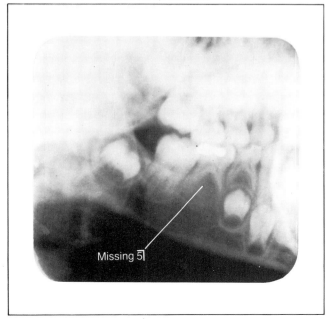

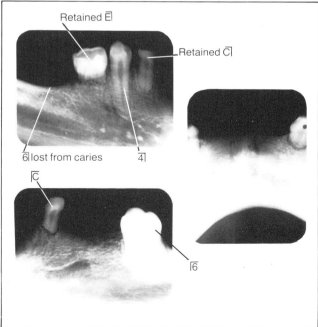

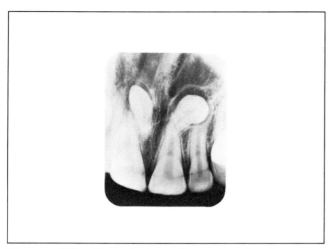

Figure 39. *Periapical radiograph showing two mesiodens, apparently inverted.*

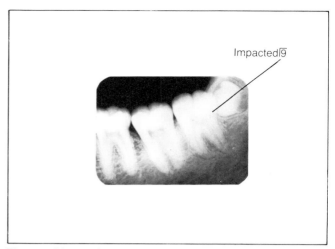

Figure 41. *Periapical radiograph showing developing lower fourth molar.*

All the teeth are larger than normal. It is, however, extremely rare.

Macrodontia of single teeth can occur and is of unknown aetiology. The tooth concerned is normal in all respects except size. Fusion and gemination, or odontomes, must not be confused with true macrodontia. An illusion of macrodontia may present when a child receives genetically the tooth size from one parent which is within the normal range, and a small jaw size from the other parent.

Microdontia of all the teeth in the dental arch is extremely rare, arising generally in cases of pituitary dwarfism. It can affect single teeth and tends to follow a familiar pattern. Some authorities include rudimentary teeth in this category, for example the 'peg' upper lateral incisors and third molars.

Congenital hemiatrophy of the jaws may present with microdontia of the affected region.

A false impression of microdontia may be gained when normal-sized teeth are set in very large jaws.

Figure 40. *Periapical radiograph showing true and supplemental upper lateral incisors preventing the eruption of 1 . One of the lateral incisors is rotated through 90°.*

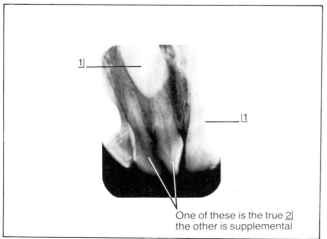

One of these is the true 2 the other is supplemental

Additional Teeth

Supernumeraries

These extra teeth, well-formed or mis-shapen, appearing singly or as multiples, are thought to arise from an extra tooth bud on the dental lamina. They may arise early to the permanent dentition of the area, with that dentition, or late to that dentition.

Supernumerary teeth forming between the maxillary central incisors are termed mesiodens. Mesiodens may erupt or fail to erupt, and frequently prevent eruption, or cause displacement of the adjacent incisor. They may appear to be inverted on periapical radiographs (Figure 39), but care must be exercised in making this interpretation due to angulation of the x-ray beam when using the bisected-angle technique. Panoramic or paralleling technique views, where the central ray is almost horizontal, sometimes show that the supernumerary is lying horizontally.

Supplemental Teeth

Radiographs play an important part in assessing the presence, number and shape of supernumeraries— especially where there is impaction or uneruption of teeth involved. Figure 40 shows 1 unerupted due to the presence of a supernumerary that has erupted into the arch. One tooth has erupted rotated through 90°, and on clinical examination it is impossible to say which tooth is the true lateral and which tooth is the supernumerary or supplemental tooth. Chronologically they have developed together.

Supplemental teeth are often found in the lower premolar region in cases of cleidocranial dysostosis. They are usually unerupted, lying in odd positions and are sometimes associated with a dentigerous cyst.

Fourth molars occasionally develop and may be either molar-form (Figure 41), or very rudimentary in nature. They are usually late to develop and could be termed late supernumeraries.

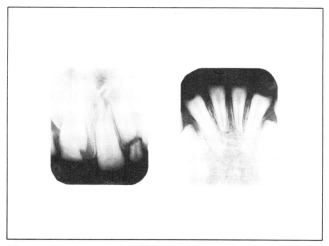

Figure 42. *Intraoral radiographic survey of a child aged 7½ years showing amelogenesis imperfecta with complete absence of enamel.*

Malformed Teeth

Amelogenesis Imperfecta

Amelogenesis imperfecta can be split into two groups:

1. Enamel hypoplasia.
2. Enamel hypocalcification.

There are occasions when teeth exhibit both forms at the same time.

In enamel hypoplasia the enamel fails to develop to normal thickness. In some cases this is a dominant mendelian characteristic which results in deficient or absent enamel in the permanent and sometimes the deciduous dentition. The dentine is usually unaffected unless extensive attrition has occurred, in which case secondary dentine may be formed.

In hypoplasia the enamel may be absent (Figure 42), smooth, or may have pitted, typically hypoplastic areas (Figure 43).

Figure 43. *Intraoral radiograph of ⌐123 region in a man aged 23 years, showing pitting of enamel in amelogenesis imperfecta.*

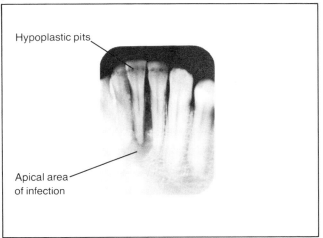

Figure 44. *Intraoral radiograph 1⌐123 region in a child of seven years suggesting hypomineralization. The enamel is of the correct thickness but is soon fractured and eroded when the teeth erupt. The unerupted teeth are complete in enamel outline, but the density of the enamel and dentine is similar.*

The enamel is not properly mineralized in enamel hypocalcification, although the correct thickness may be produced (Figure 44). Radiographically this enamel has much the same density as the dentine, and it is hard to determine the line of junction between the two materials.

Dentinogenesis Imperfecta

Also termed hereditary opalescent dentine (Figure 45), dentinogenesis imperfecta is a dominant hereditary characteristic which does not appear to be sex-linked. Both dentitions are involved. There is early partial or total obliteration of the pulp chambers and root canals by continuous formation of dentine. Because of the absence of the radiolucent pulpal shadow the dentine appears to be more opaque than normal to the eye,

Figure 45. *Dentinogenesis imperfecta in a boy of 15 years. The pulps have calcified and there is no sign of enamel remaining. ⌐1 has a jacket crown and 2⌐ a metal-backed crown.*

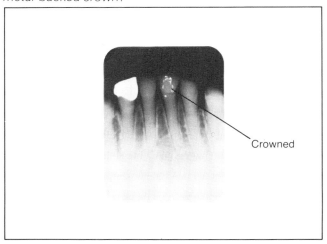

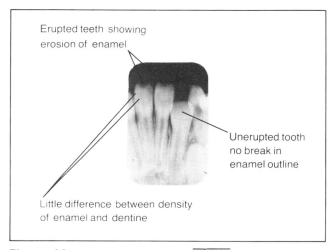

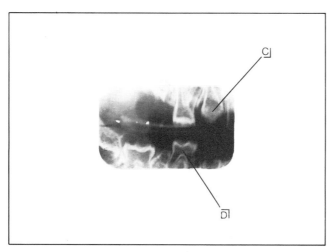

Figure 46. *Right bitewing radiograph showing shell teeth in the deciduous dentition of a child aged two years.*

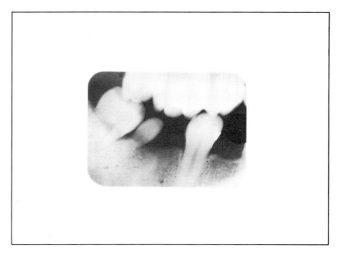

Figure 48. *Right bitewing radiograph showing possible rudimentary 7⏌. This could, however, be a supernumerary —if both 76⏋ have been extracted.*

though it is, in fact, more radiolucent. The roots of the teeth are often shorter than usual, though the surrounding tissues are normal.

Lack of the scalloped amelodentinal junction is probably responsible for early loss of the enamel. The latter fractures away easily and rapid attrition of the exposed soft dentine follows.

Shell Teeth

There is a reduced number of tubules in the dentine of shell teeth, and in some cases the teeth may appear to be almost entirely composed of enamel (Figure 46). The

Figure 47. *Part of a Panelipse radiograph showing rudimentary ⏊8 no longer supported by bone. A dense bone island is evident at the mesial apex ⏋6. An intraoral radiograph is necessary to make a differential diagnosis with sclerosing osteitis.*

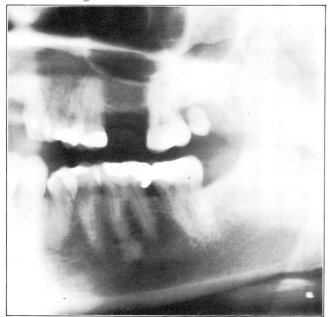

enclosed pulp chambers do not calcify and, as yet, the condition has not been shown to be hereditary. It is a very rare condition.

Rudimentary Teeth

Rudimentary teeth can be considered a form of microdontia, though it is probably better to describe them separately as they do not follow the pattern of the normal teeth in the region. They are often peg-like, and are most frequently found in the upper lateral incisor and upper third molar regions (Figure 47). Supernumerary teeth are often peg-shaped, too, and it is impossible at times to tell whether a tooth is rudimentary or supernumerary (Figure 48), especially when there have been extractions in the area.

Fusion, Concrescence and Gemination

Fusion results when two tooth germs approximate, the dentine of both teeth becoming involved in the process.

Figure 49. *Intraoral radiograph ⏋78 region in a woman aged 32 showing true fusion of ⏋78.*

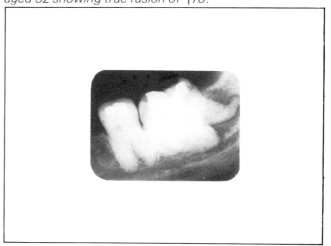

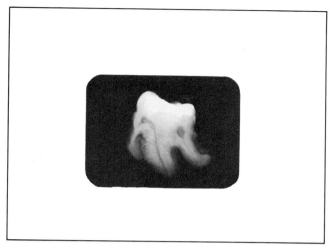

Figure 50. *Radiograph of extracted $\overline{78}$ from Figure 49 showing the pulps of these teeth clearly. The pulps do not appear to be united at all.*

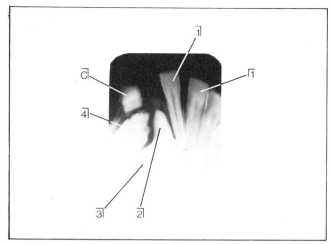

Figure 52. *Periapical radiograph showing $\overline{432}$. $\overline{4}$ was related to an abscess on $\overline{D}$, and appears to be hypoplastic.*

Whether fusion is complete or partial depends on the stage of development of the two teeth at the point of fusion. In cases of early fusion the teeth involved may become united to form one very large tooth (Figures 49 and 50) (not to be confused with macrodontia). In cases of later fusion there may only be union of the roots.

Concrescence is the bonding together of two or more teeth by cementum. Care is required in extraction of upper molars in these cases as there is always the possibility of fracture of the maxillary tuberosity. This also applies in the case of true fusion described above.

Gemination arises when a tooth germ splits, generally resulting in a tooth with two crowns and a single root (Figure 51). The condition is found in both dentitions—sometimes in the same individual.

It may not be possible to differentiate between gemination and fusion when a normal and supernumerary tooth are involved.

Turner Tooth

Infection at the apices or bifurcation of a deciduous molar can result in hypoplasia of the crown of the permanent successor. This is due to the follicle of the latter becoming involved in the infective process. Figure 52 is an example of a Turner tooth before eruption, the deciduous first molar having been lost as the result of an abscess. Radiographically the hypoplasia presents as an irregularity of the enamel surface.

Taurodont Teeth

These odd-shaped teeth (Figure 53) can be seen in the skulls of Neanderthal man. Occasionally they appear in

Figure 53. *An orthopantomogram showing oligodontia in a boy of nine years. Two large invaginated odontomes are erupting into the upper arch, and only one or two further upper teeth are developing to follow the few remaining deciduous teeth. $\overline{6E}$ are taurodont and small compared with $\underline{E6}$. He had other developmental defects, including reduced size of the right side of his body, skull and right hand.*

Figure 51. *Intraoral radiograph of a girl of 14 years showing gemination of the crown of $\underline{2}$.*

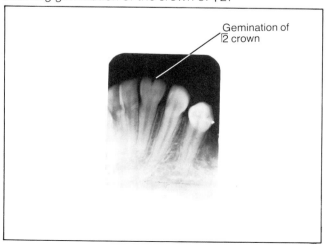

Gemination of
$\underline{2}$ crown

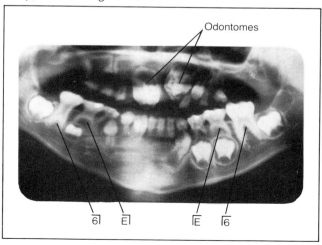

Odontomes

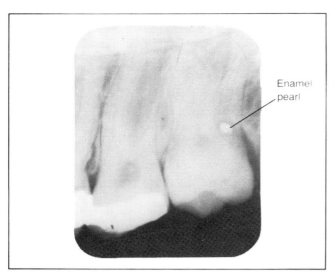

Figure 54. *Periapical radiograph showing enamel pearl near root bifurcation of* ⌊8.

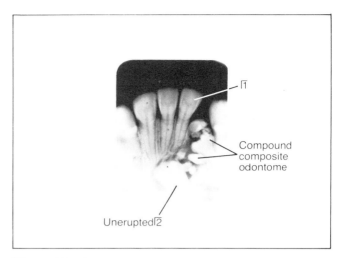

Figure 56. *Compound composite odontome in a girl of 15 years, which has prevented the eruption of* ⌐2. *The separate denticles are quite obvious.*

the dentition of modern man, suggesting the expression of some genes derived from the Neanderthals.

Such teeth are characterized by having long bodies, large pulp chambers and small roots (Figure 53).

In marked degrees of taurodontism the body of the tooth consists of a thick trunk ending in a concave surface surrounded by two or three short webbed roots.

Odontomes

Enamel Pearl

The enamel pearl, or nodule, is most frequently found at the junction of the roots of the maxillary molar

Figure 55. *Complex odontome in a man of 29 years, closely related to an unerupted* ⌐8. *The occlusal radiograph (not shown) confirms that this is a mass of tissue rather than separate denticles.*

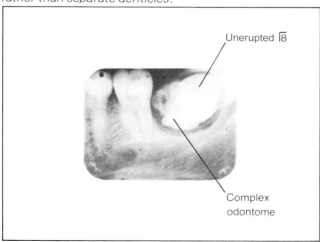

(Figure 54). It is a small mass of enamel fixed to the tooth and has been known to contain dentine and occasionally a small strand of pulp continuous with the main pulp chamber.

It is not a common condition and does not appear to arise from teeth in the incisor region.

Radiographically a differential diagnosis has to be made with calculus on the teeth, and a salivary calculus related to the parotid duct or gland. Clinical examination of the area will show the presence of calculus on the teeth or the presence of the enamel pearl, and radiographs taken at different angulations will assist in the diagnosis of salivary calculus.

Complex Composite Odontome

A complex composite odontome is a tumour composed of more than one type of dental tissue, and bearing no similarity to a normal tooth. The calcified material is laid down as an irregular mass surrounded by a capsule similar to the tooth follicle.

A complex odontome may be present in any part of the tooth-bearing areas of the dental arches.

Radiographically it presents as an irregular mass of radio-opaque material surrounded by a radiolucent band, and is frequently associated with unerupted teeth or supernumeraries (Figure 55).

Compound Composite Odontome

The compound odontome differs from the complex odontome in that it is built up of multiple denticles clumped together (Figure 56), in many cases the denticles appearing to be rudimentary teeth. They are enclosed in a radiolucent area bounded by a radio-opaque border, again resembling a tooth follicle.

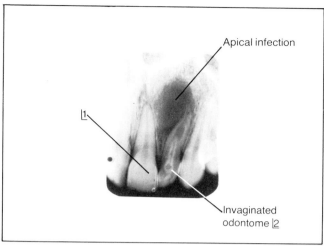

Figure 57. *Periapical radiograph of ⌊2 region in a girl of 19 years of age, showing erupted invaginated odontome with a periapical area. The enamel inside the tooth is quite obvious and the radiographic appearance is diagnostic of the condition.*

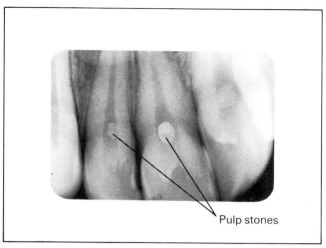

Figure 58. *Periapical radiograph showing pulp stones in 321 ⌊1 in a boy of 14 years.*

Invaginated Odontome

Invaginated odontomes sometimes termed 'dens in dente' are not 'teeth within teeth', but are formed by an infolding of the enamel organ. The result is the production of enamel within the body of the tooth (Figure 57). In a normal-looking tooth the infolding is generally at the cingulum and is not readily evident on clinical examination. The invagination allows debris to collect inside the tooth, and being very close to the pulp in many cases there is early exposure followed by periapical infection.

Radiography of these odontomes, preferably before eruption, is important. Forewarned, the practitioner can fill the cingulum on eruption of the tooth and prevent a periapical area from developing. The radiographic appearance is diagnostic of the condition.

Not all invaginated odontomes, which usually occur in the upper incisor region, are tooth-like and extraction may be indicated.

Pulp Stones

The incidence of pulp stones is greater than might be expected, and has been quoted as high as 50 per cent. Radiographically they present as round or oval opaque bodies of varying sizes, partly obliterating the pulp chambers and canals (Figure 58). They may be single or multiple, and do not appear to be related to any particular disease or trauma process. Some may not be visible on radiographs.

Where these pulp calcifications arise early on in the life of the tooth the pulp chamber will maintain its original outline, not demonstrating the changes anticipated with age.

Pulp stones can sometimes be seen in unerupted teeth.

Bone Abnormalities

Tori

Bony exostoses can occur on the surface of the maxilla or mandible. Usually they are evident on the lingual aspect of the mandible in the premolar or molar regions, unilaterally or bilaterally, and are termed tori mandibularis (Figure 59).

Tori of the palate generally occur in the midline of the hard palate. These very hard areas can cause problems in the construction of dentures.

Tori present radiographically as radio-opaque areas on lateral views, and are differentiated from odontomes by the fact that there are no radiolucent capsules surrounding them. In the mandible an occlusal view will eliminate the likelihood of submandibular calculus.

Figure 59. *Occlusal view ⌈78 region in a 40-year-old woman showing bony exostosis opposite the molars lingually.*

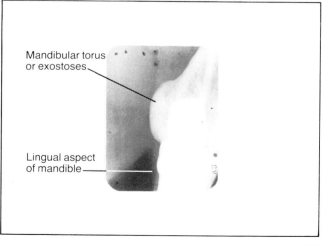

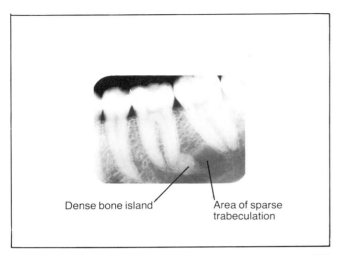

Dense bone island   Area of sparse
                           trabeculation

Figure 60. *Dense bone islands at the distal apex of ⌐6. These bone abnormalities frequently present in this region.*

Dense Bone Islands

Dense bone islands are generally an incidental finding on dental radiographs, and present as small or large radio-opaque areas, usually situated at the apical region of the lower first molars (Figure 60). The radio-opacity is continuous with the lamina dura of the socket and the periodontal membrane is depicted as quite normal on the radiograph. This helps to differentiate the condition from sclerosing osteitis resulting from infection or trauma, where changes in the periodontal membrane shadows on radiographs are to be expected. There is no surrounding capsule to a dense bone island, so differential diagnosis with odontome is straightforward.

An occlusal radiograph will demonstrate that the opacity is within the mandible, and eliminate the possibility of exostosis or submandibular calculus.

Cleft Palate

The condition of cleft palate results from complete or partial failure of the facial processes to unite and can be

Figure 61. *Left alveolar and palatal cleft in 25-year-old man. ⌐2 is missing.*

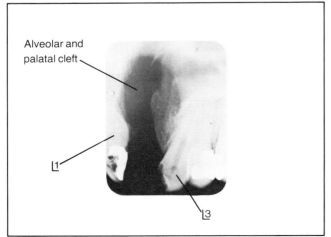

Alveolar and
palatal cleft

L1

L3

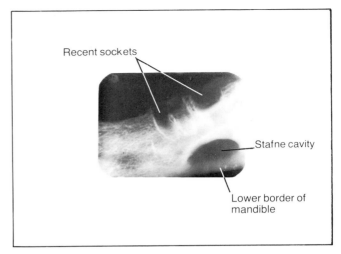

Recent sockets

Stafne cavity

Lower border of
mandible

Figure 62. *Stafne cavity at lower border of left mandible. There are recent sockets evident. The idiopathic bone cavity was an incidental finding.*

genetically significant. Cleft palates may be unilateral or bilateral and can be shown radiographically (Figure 61).

Often the teeth related to the cleft are distorted, peg-like or missing. There may be supernumeraries evident and teeth in the area may be buried or partly erupted into the cleft. The lateral incisor is often absent.

Stafne (1958) reports a small median alveolar cleft of the maxilla which is extremely rare. These are said to arise as a result of non-union of the two centres of calcification of the globular process.

Idiopathic Bone Cavities

These radiolucent areas, sometimes called Stafne cavities, are generally related to the lower half of the body of the mandible in the molar region (Figure 62). They are nearly always an incidental finding and symptomless.

They appear as round or oval radiolucencies and may involve the lower border of the mandible. When their surrounding cortex is continuous with that of the mandibular cortex they create the impression that they are not enclosed cavities, but are depressions in the mandible. Those cases that have been investigated show the contents of the deficiency to be in some cases connective tissue, and in others an enclosed lobe of the submandibular salivary gland.

Being part of the mandibular cortex the surrounding outline of these cavities is usually more dense than that depicted by a developing cyst. Differential diagnosis also has to be made with non-epithelialized bone cyst.

Unerupted Teeth

Failure of teeth to erupt can be the result of localized or generalized crowding. The overcrowding may be due to underdevelopment of part of or the complete dental arch, or it may arise as a result of large teeth taking up too much room in a normal-sized arch. In many cases impaction and misplacement of teeth will result.

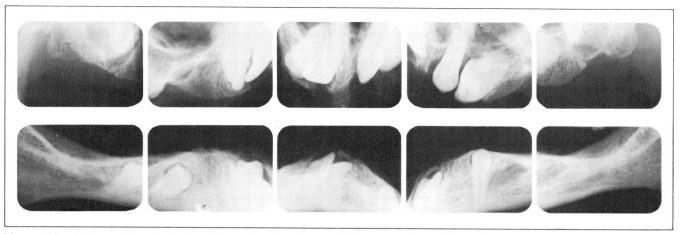

Figure 63. *Full-mouth periapical radiographs showing multiple uneruption of anterior teeth in a man aged 52 years. The tooth in ⌊4 region is abnormal in shape and no molars are evident. There are no other signs of systemic disturbance.*

Multiple Unerupted Teeth

Multiple unerupted teeth occur in such conditions as hypoparathyroidism and cleidocranial dysostosis, though sometimes there may be no evidence of any underlying systemic disease. On occasions there are hereditary factors involved.

Figure 63 shows a set of full-mouth intraoral radiographs of a man aged 52 years showing buried teeth anteriorly and no sign of any molar teeth. There was no skeletal suggestion of cleidocranial dysostosis or other systemic disturbance. The tooth in ⌊4 region appears to be an odontome.

Single Unerupted Teeth

Single unerupted teeth are common and may be due to a variety of causes, such as overcrowding of the arch, infection or retention of a deciduous predecessor, displacement of the tooth germ, early loss of a deciduous molar, or presence of dentigerous cyst, tumour, alveolar cleft or supernumerary. About 75 per cent of supernumerary teeth are unerupted.

Impacted Teeth

Teeth that have some structure wholly or partly preventing their eruption are termed impacted teeth. Lack of space due to overcrowding is the most likely cause of this condition. Rotation of the tooth bud is thought to be another common cause of impaction, but this may be related to the overcrowding. The teeth most frequently involved are the third molars.

Third Molars

Lower Third Molars

The mandibular third molar is the most commonly unerupted and impacted tooth of the permanent dentition. Modern man's diet has been refined to such an extent that most of the fibrous roughage has been removed, and this may be largely responsible for the underdevelopment of the jaws—a feature of modern development! The third molar being the last tooth to erupt is therefore short of space, and the teenage patient attending the general practitioner with an impacted molar and pericoronal infection in this region is a frequent sight.

The lower third molar can take up a number of positions when impacted, some of which are illustrated in Figures 64 to 69. Difficulty of removal of these teeth is assessed by the condition of the surrounding bone, the depth of the teeth in the bone, their angulation, the size, shape and number of their roots, and the proximity of the roots to the inferior dental canal.

The angulation of the impacted tooth is assessed with respect to the normal occlusal plane.

Figure 64 shows a mesioangular impaction of 8⌋, the most common form of impaction of lower third molars.

Figure 64. *Periapical radiograph 8⌋ of a woman aged 35 years showing mesioangular impaction. The crown is covered with bone distally, the roots are fused, and the inferior dental canal appears to groove the roots as the lamina is thinned in this region.*

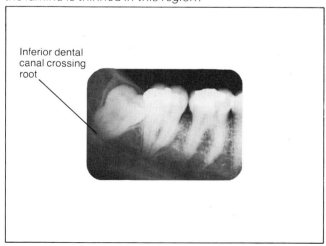

Inferior dental canal crossing root

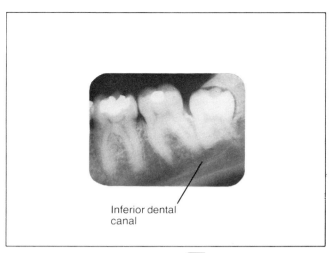

Inferior dental
canal

Figure 65. *Vertically impacted $\lceil 8$. The crown is almost completely covered in bone and there are two roots. Relative to the occlusal plane there is a slight distal tilt.*

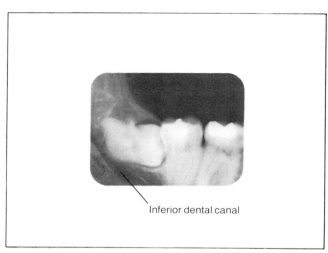

Inferior dental canal

Figure 67. *Horizontal $\overline{8\rceil}$ in a man of 31 years with two roots possibly close to roof of inferior dental canal. The crown is covered by bone and close to $\overline{7\rceil}$. There is no sign of resorption of either tooth.*

Other possible impactions are:

1. Vertical (Figure 65). The bone of the ramus prevents eruption of the third molar into the arch. Sometimes the anterior cusps can be seen clinically in these impactions, and food stagnation areas are common, leading to pericoronitis.

2. Distoangular (Figure 66). The crown of the tooth points distally into the ramus and is often completely buried in the bone.

3. Horizontal. Several forms of horizontal impaction can arise. The most common occurs with the crown lying mesially towards the distal root of the lower second molar (Figure 67), the depth of the tooth in the bone to a large extent determining the difficulty of its removal.

Another type of horizontal impaction is where the crown faces distally and the roots mesially. This is not a frequent occurrence in the mandible, but is quite common with the upper third molar.

A laterally-lying horizontally impacted tooth is termed a transverse impaction. Again, the crown can be in either of two positions, the occlusal surface facing either buccally or lingually (Figure 68a). An occlusal radiograph is necessary with this type of impaction to determine exactly the position of the crown. A standard-sized periapical film is quite adequate for this assessment and is very helpful prior to surgery. Figures 68a and b show periapical and occlusal views of transverse $\overline{8\rceil}$ with the crown facing lingually.

4. Inversion of third molars can occur (Figure 69) though this is not a frequent occurrence and is usually related to the presence of a dentigerous cyst.

Figure 66. *Distoangular $\overline{8\rceil}$ with fused root, the crown pointing up into the ramus and covered in bone. The mandibular canal is not related to the apex.*

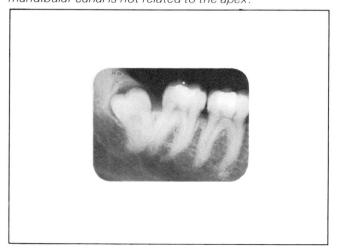

Figure 68 (a). *Transverse impaction of $\overline{8\rceil}$. It is necessary to have an occlusal radiograph to determine in which direction the crown is pointing. **(b)** Occlusal radiograph $\overline{8\rceil}$ shows that the crown is facing lingually. This particular film does not give any indication of root formation or number due to its obliquity.*

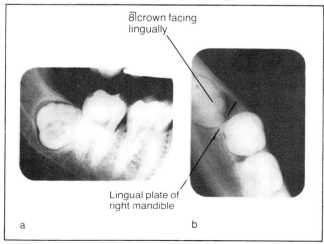

$\overline{8}$crown facing
lingually

Lingual plate of
right mandible

a   b

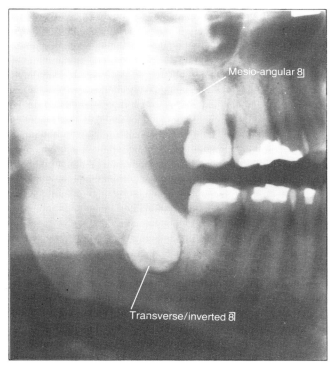

Figure 69. *Part of a Panelipse radiograph showing inverted* $\overline{8|}$ *in a man of 44 years.* $\underline{8|}$ *is impacted mesioangularly against* $\overline{7|}$ *.*

Upper Third Molars

The impactions already discussed can involve the maxillary third molar, and Figure 70 shows a mesioangular $\underline{8|}$.

Figure 71 illustrates a distoangular $\lfloor 8$; Figure 72 a horizontal $\underline{8|}$ on a Panorex radiograph with the crown facing distally; and Figure 73 a horizontally impacted $\lfloor 8$ with the crown facing mesially and preventing eruption of $\lfloor 7$.

Figure 70. *Mesioangular impaction of* $8|$ *in a woman of 26 years. The tooth has conical roots and there is plenty of room for the tooth to have erupted into the arch.*

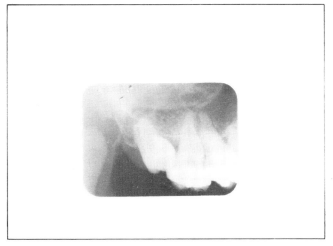

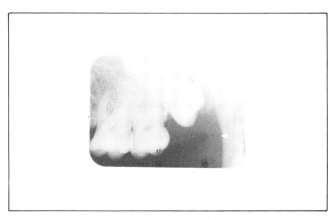

Figure 71. *Distoangular impaction* $\lfloor 8$ *with fused roots.*

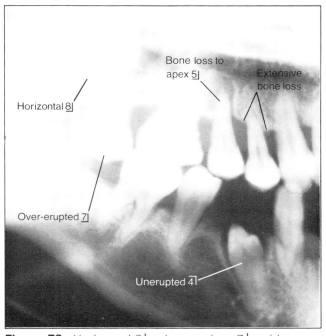

Figure 72. *Horizontal* $\underline{8|}$ *, above apices* $\underline{7|}$ *, with crown facing distally in part of a Panorex radiograph. Unerupted* $\overline{4|}$ *is also evident and generalized extensive bone loss.*

Figure 73. *Horizontal* $\lfloor 8$ *crown facing mesially, impacted against and preventing full eruption of* $\lfloor 7$ *into the arch of a man of 31 years.*

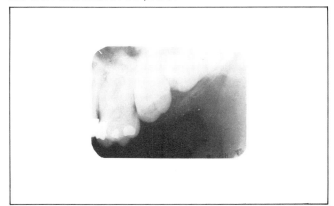

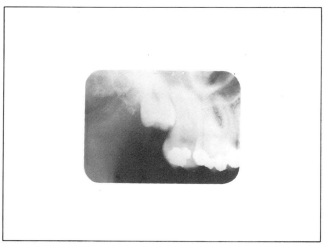

Figure 74. *Vertical 8| impacted against bulge of crown of 7| in the same patient as Figure 73.*

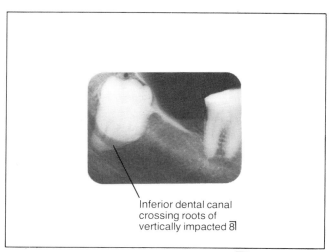

Inferior dental canal crossing roots of vertically impacted 8|

Figure 76. *Roots of vertically impacted 8| appear to be grooved by the inferior dental canal. The patient is 60 years of age.*

In Figure 74 8| is impacted against 7| vertically in a man aged 31 years. His other third molars are impacted horizontally (not shown).

The lateral skull view (Figure 75) shows inverted |8, which is possibly related to a cyst.

Figure 75. *True lateral skull view of a girl aged 19 years showing inverted |8. This type of third molar inversion is generally related to a dentigerous cyst. The crown of another molar is evident further anteriorly and high up in the maxilla.*

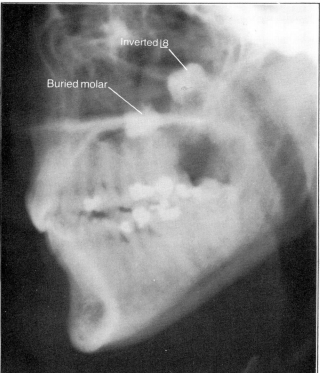

Inverted |8

Buried molar

Relationship of Mandibular Third Molars to the Inferior Dental Canal

It has already been mentioned that an occlusal view of the lower impacted wisdom tooth is helpful in determining the position of the crown buccolingually. Another important item is assessment of the proximity of the inferior dental canal to the roots of the impacted tooth. Root formation and number vary considerably in lower third molars and they have been known to encircle the canal completely. Constriction of both the root and

Figure 77. *Mesioangular 8| with roots bent and running along the upper border and to one side of the canal. There are two retained roots of 7| evident. The patient is 31 years of age.*

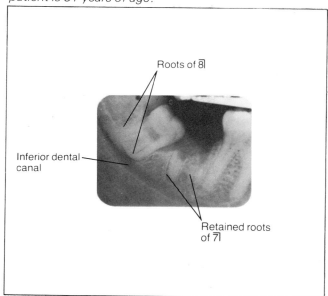

Roots of 8|

Inferior dental canal

Retained roots of 7|

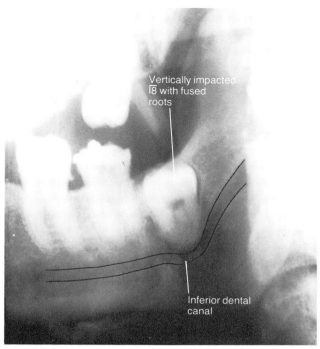

Figure 78. *Vertically impacted ⌐8 in a woman aged 46 years. The developing roots have pushed the inferior dental canal downwards.*

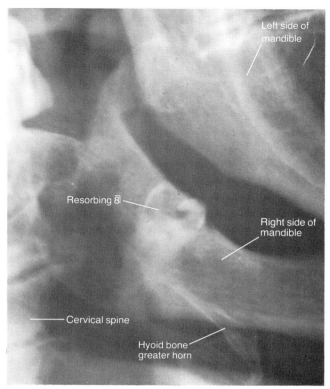

Figure 79. *Part of oblique lateral radiograph of a woman aged 54 years. The crown of unerupted 8⌐ is undergoing resorption.*

the canal on the radiograph may indicate this condition.

More often the roots are grooved by the canal lying directly alongside (Figure 76), or in their development the roots are bent and run above and parallel to the canal (Figure 77). Sometimes the canal is depressed by the roots (Figure 78).

Absence of the lamina dura of the socket crossing the canal or absence of the upper or lower borders of the canal itself indicate a close relationship of the tooth and canal. In all cases careful radiographic interpretation will pay dividends when surgery is undertaken.

Parallax views, discussed later in the section on unerupted canines (page 27), will give an indication of the nearness of the inferior dental canal to the unerupted molar.

Resorption

Impacted third molars sometimes undergo resorption (Figure 79), and on occasions they will cause resorption of the teeth against which they are impacted (Figure 80).

In the case of the resorbing impacted teeth enamel and dentine may be resorbed until a 'ghost' shell is all that remains. On other occasions there may be only irregular superficial resorption.

If transplantation of third molars is being considered a good preoperative radiograph of the tooth concerned is necessary to ensure that there has been no resorption of the crown enamel.

Second Molars

Second molars seldom fail to erupt, though occasionally the lower second molar may be unerupted or impacted.

The most common impactions are:

1. Where the lower second molar has a mesioangular or horizontal inclination and the third molar has erupted over it—usually with a steep mesial tilt (Figure 81a).

Figure 80. *Low mesioangular 8⌐ with conical root. Considerable resorption of both roots of 7⌐ has taken place.*

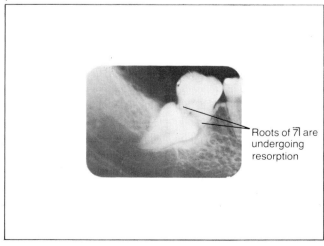

Roots of 7⌐ are undergoing resorption

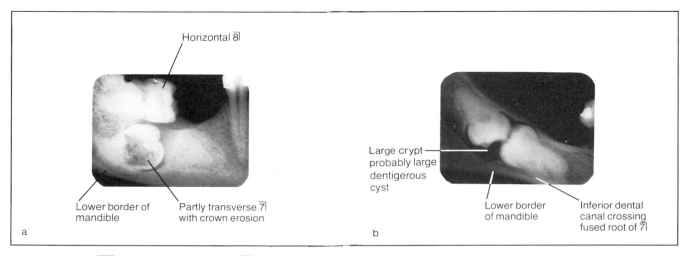

Horizontal $\overline{8|}$

Lower border of mandible

Partly transverse $\overline{7|}$ with crown erosion

Large crypt probably large dentigerous cyst

Lower border of mandible

Inferior dental canal crossing fused root of $\overline{7|}$

a

b

Figure 81 (a). *$\overline{87|}$ are both horizontal, $\overline{7|}$ having taken up a slightly transverse position. There is a pocket leading down to the crown of $\overline{7|}$. The crown of $\overline{7|}$ may be carious or resorbing.* **(b)** *Crown to crown impaction of $\overline{87|}$ in a woman aged 54 years. The crypt of $\overline{8|}$ appears unnaturally large and may well, at this stage, be a dentigerous cyst. The mandibular canal crosses the roots of horizontal $\overline{7|}$.*

2. Where the occlusal surfaces of the crowns of the second and third molars are impacted together (Figure 81b).

Other forms of impaction of second molars occur but they are rare.

First Molars

The reason for uneruption or impaction of first molars is somewhat obscure, though the presence of dentigerous cyst is one possibility. Eruption and impaction problems can occur with all three molars at the same time.

Figure 82 illustrates what may have been a submerged $\overline{|6}$ impacted beneath $\overline{|57}$.

Premolars

It is almost always the second premolar that fails to erupt into the arch. The first premolar usually manages to get into position at the expense of either the canine or the second premolar. Occasionally the crown of the first premolar will be pushed out buccally to the arch.

The reasons for non-eruption and impaction of the second premolar are early loss of the second deciduous molar, the first permanent molar tilting forwards into the space, and large teeth in small arches.

Figure 82. *Vertically impacted $\overline{|6}$ in a man of 21 years. The crowns of $\overline{|57}$ have tilted into the space above $\overline{|6}$ leaving no room for the eruption of this tooth.*

Figure 83. *Palatally buried $\underline{|5}$.*

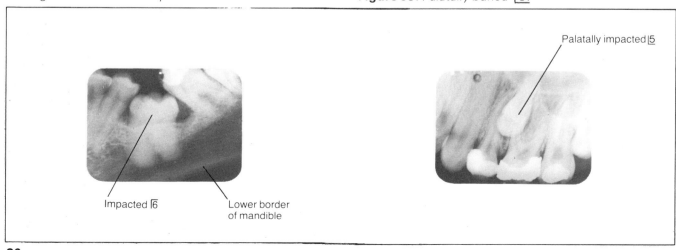

Impacted $\overline{|6}$

Lower border of mandible

Palatally impacted $|5$

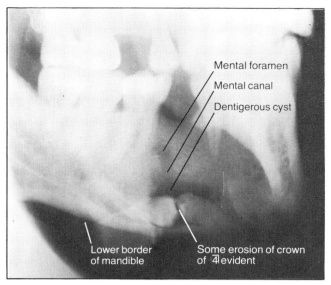

Figure 84. *Horizontal crown to crown impaction of $\overline{54|}$ with teeth near the lower border of the mandible. There is a large radiolucency related to the crowns of these teeth and this may be cystic in nature. The mental canal and foramen are also evident, though this could just be a sinus from the 'cystic' area. A second intraoral film would help in the differential diagnosis.*

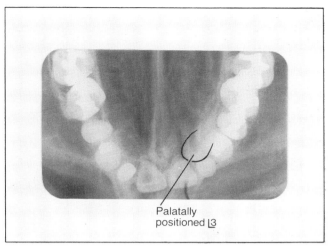

Palatally positioned |3

Figure 85. *Vertex occlusal radiograph with the central ray passing down the long axis of the upper anterior teeth showing |3 palatally placed.*

Most upper impacted premolars have their crowns palatally inclined, and some erupt in this position. They may, however, remain completely buried and impacted (Figure 83).

Lower premolars tend to erupt lingually when there is a shortage of room in the arch. They may remain buried and quite frequently end up occupying a horizontal position low down in the body of the mandible (Figure 84).

The mental foramen may be a problem in dealing with this type of impaction and its position should be accurately ascertained when surgery is undertaken.

Canines

Upper Canines

The second most frequently impacted tooth is the upper canine. On occasions it will not come down into the arch even when there is sufficient room. In these instances the deciduous canines may remain in place.

The unerupted teeth can take up a number of positions, and the crowns may be buccal or palatal to the arch. In the vast majority of cases they appear to lie palatally and fail to erupt.

Before considering a treatment plan it is necessary to know the position of these teeth as this may determine whether extraction, exposure of the crown for traction or eruption purposes, or in some instances transplantation is to be undertaken.

Localization of upper canines. A vertex occlusal radiograph (Figure 85) will show whether an upper canine is buccal or palatal to the arch, but this radiographic view has several disadvantages:

1. The film is screen film exposed in a cassette, hence some detail is lost.

2. If the central ray is projected through the frontal bone the canine will not be seen through the opacity. The central ray must be projected through the true vertex of the skull down the long axis of the upper anteriors.

3. Even in a cassette the exposure to the patient is considerable, and repeat films are often necessary, thereby doubling the dose.

A true lateral and a posteroanterior view of the skull may well settle the problem of the position of the teeth under consideration, and there is the added advantage that the two radiographic views are at 90° to each other. On a number of occasions, however, it is very hard to see the unerupted tooth or teeth satisfactorily on these views and accurate assessment is not possible.

The method of using parallax to determine whether the crowns of the impacted teeth are buccal or palatal to the arch is straightforward once the fundamental geometry is understood.

Two methods of using this technique are considered here, both of which can be satisfactorily employed in general practice. The first method uses standard periapical films, and the second the panoramic film taken with a Panorex (orbiting panoramic) machine.

Localization of buried teeth by parallax using intraoral films. Buccal or palatal position of canines, supernumeraries and odontomes relative to the arch can be determined, as can the relative nearness of the inferior dental canal to third molar teeth.

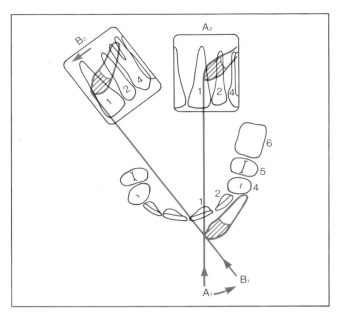

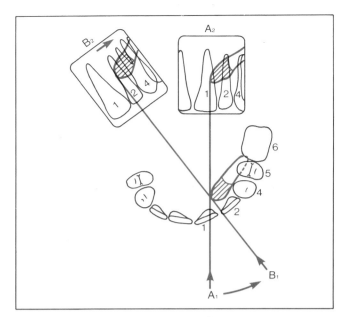

Figure 86. *Buccally positioned |3. When the X-ray tubehead moves from position A1 back to position B1 the image of |3 crown moves from over |2 to over |1 on the intraoral radiographs represented by A2 and B2. So for teeth positioned buccally to the arch, when the tubehead moves back, their image appears to move forwards.*

Figure 88. *Palatally positioned |3. When the X-ray tubehead moves from position A1 back to position B1 the image of the tip of |3 crown moves from over |1 to over |2 on the intraoral radiographs represented by A2 and B2. So for teeth positioned palatally to the arch, when the tubehead moves back their image appears to move back with the tubehead.*

Figure 87. *Standard occlusal radiograph centred on 1|1, and periapical radiograph centred on |3 region. The upper left canine appears to have moved in the opposite direction to the tubehead and is therefore buccally positioned to the arch.*

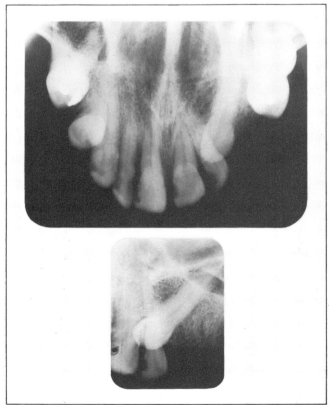

In Figure 86 the buried canine is buccal to the arch. In the lower part of the diagram A1 represents the position of the tubehead and A2 the resulting periapical radiograph.

If the tubehead is now moved to position B1, the resulting radiograph will be B2.

It can be seen that the crown of the canine appears to have moved forwards whilst the x-ray tubehead has moved backwards.

Hence for buccal positions to the arch the buried tooth appears to move in the *opposite* direction to the x-ray tubehead (Figure 87).

In Figure 88 the buried canine is palatal to the arch. A2 represents the radiographic appearance when the tubehead is at position A1. B2 represents the radiographic appearance when the tubehead is moved backwards to position B1. The image of the canine appears to move in the same direction as the tubehead.

Hence for palatal positions to the arch the buried tooth appears to move in the *same* direction as the tubehead.

To determine the position of upper canines if *both* are unerupted in the same jaw, a standard occlusal radiographic view and one periapical view of each canine are required (Figure 89).

Localization of unerupted anterior teeth using the Panorex. The position of teeth, supernumeraries and odontomes near the midline can be determined using the Panorex, an orbiting panoramic machine with two centres of rotation. There is a tube shift between the

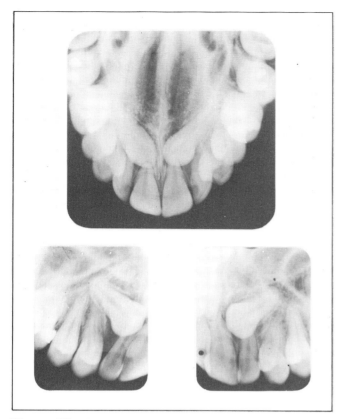

Figure 89. *Standard occlusal radiograph centred on 1|1, and periapical radiographs centred on 3|3. The unerupted upper canines appear to have moved with the tubehead and are therefore both palatally positioned with respect to the arch.*

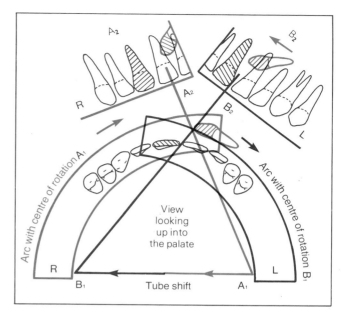

Figure 90. *Diagrammatic representation of parallax using a Panorex panoramic radiograph and considering a buccally placed canine (see the text for explanation).*

exposures for the left and right jaws, and the anterior region from canine to canine is seen on both exposures.

This can be represented diagrammatically as in Figure 90. The lower part of the diagram is a plan view looking up into the upper dental arch. A1 and B1 are the two centres of rotation of the x-ray beam. The beam rotating about A1 covers the trough of the patient's right side (marked in red) right round to |2 region. The centre of rotation then moves over to B1, and the beam covers the trough of the patient's left side (marked in black) from the 2| region round to |8.

The blank area of film in the middle of every Panorex radiograph has been omitted for simplicity.

A2 and B2 show the resulting radiographic appearances (diagrammatically) from centres of rotation A1 and B1, respectively.

It can be seen that the image of the buccally-positioned canine, considering first A2 then B2, moves towards the patient's right as shown by the red arrow on B2.

Great care must be made in this assessment, particularly with respect to which film results from which

centre of rotation. A diagram to hand is of great assistance.

In Figure 91 the unerupted canine is palatally placed. Considering first A2 then B2, the palatally placed canine appears to move to the patient's left, as shown by the red arrow in B2.

Figure 91. *Diagrammatic representation of parallax using a Panorex panoramic radiograph and considering a palatally placed canine (see text for explanation).*

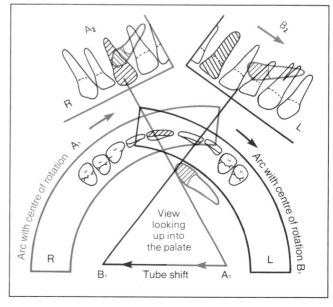

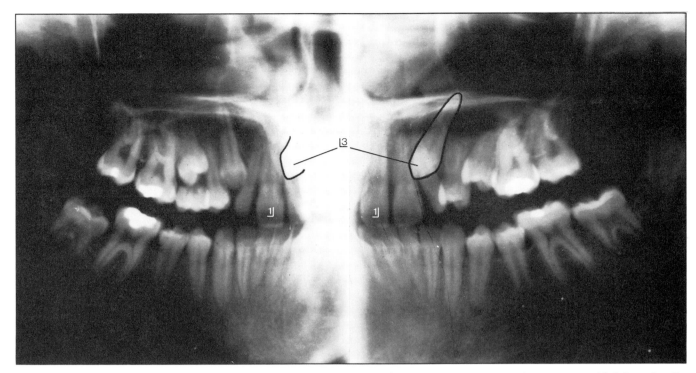

Figure 92. *Panorex radiograph. Using the diagram in Figure 91 it can be seen that the unerupted ⌊3 is palatally positioned. Considering first the patient's right side, then the patient's left side, ⌊3 appears to have moved to the patient's left.*

Relate Figure 91 to Figure 92 which illustrates a palatally positioned⌊3.

Lower Canines

Unerupted lower canines take up a variety of positions. Impaction of the mandibular canine is unusual. They are sometimes found to be deep in the mandible, generally with their crowns pointing towards the midline.

Figure 93. *Odontome in 2⌋ region preventing eruption of upper right lateral incisor.*

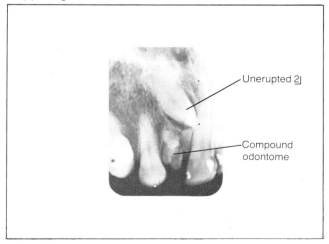

Incisors

Uneruption and impaction of incisors can occur in overcrowding, the lateral incisor usually being the tooth affected since it erupts after the central incisor.

The presence of supernumeraries (e.g. mesiodens and supplementals) and odontomes may prevent the eruption of incisors, radiographs providing the diagnosis in such cases.

Figure 93 illustrates 2⌋ unable to erupt into the arch because of the presence of an odontome.

Misplacement of Teeth

To a large extent this topic has already been covered in the sections on eruption and impaction of teeth, but five additional conditions should be considered:

1. Wandering teeth.
2. Effect of cysts.
3. Transposition.
4. Transplantation.
5. Submerged teeth.

Wandering Teeth

Teeth appear to have the ability to move considerable distances for no apparent reason, and there have been instances of a lower canine moving across the midline to the other side of the mandible (Stafne 1958). Premolars

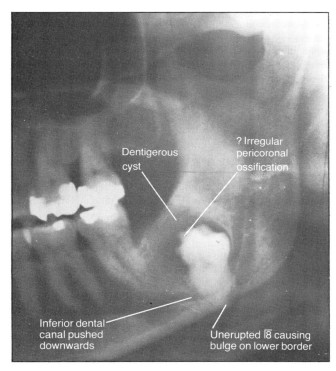

Figure 94. *Part of Panelipse radiograph showing dentigerous cyst on ⌐8. The tooth has been depressed to the lower border of the mandible taking the inferior dental canal with it. There is some irregular ossification evident.*

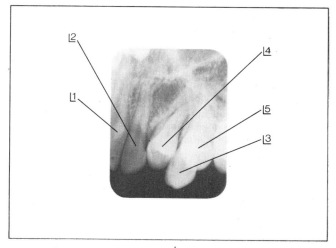

Figure 95. *Transposition of ⌐34 in a boy aged 12 years (note position of the apices). In addition there is overcrowding in this quadrant.*

also frequently migrate, and it would appear that this movement is always in the direction in which the crown points. Premolars found near the lower border of the mandible may well be supplemental teeth that have been unable to erupt into the fully-occupied arch.

Effect of Cysts

Whilst radicular dental cysts can push the roots of erupted teeth apart, the dentigerous cyst is often the cause of considerable displacement of a whole tooth or teeth. Upper third molars are found under the orbit, and lower third molars can be pushed downwards until the roots depress the lower border of the mandible (Figure 94). Any tooth can be affected, and it is interesting to note that badly displaced teeth can find their way back into the arch once the cyst has been treated successfully.

Transposition of Teeth

Transposition of teeth is not a frequent anomaly. When it does occur it is usually the upper canine and the first premolar that are transposed (Figure 95), and the condition can present bilaterally.

Should the first premolar have a large palatal cusp and be unsightly, the treatment of choice may well be to stone this cusp down over a period of several years.

Transplantation

Although it is not a developmental abnormality transplantation of teeth is considered here. Figure 96 shows a developing 8⌐ that has been removed and transplanted into the socket of ⌐6, the latter having been extracted following periapical infection. The radiograph was taken eight months after the operation and shows some root resorption. It also shows the transplanted tooth a little below the occlusal plane which, although normal at the time of operation, suggests possible ankylosis is still evident some time later.

Submerged Teeth

It has been suggested that the submerged appearance of the retained deciduous second molar is due to the fact

Figure 96. *Transplantation of 8⌐ to ⌐6 socket in a girl of 16 years. The radiograph shows some resorption of the roots eight months after the operation.*

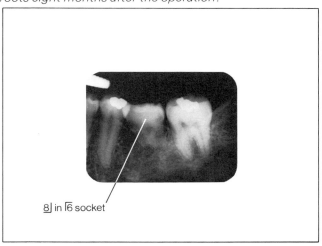

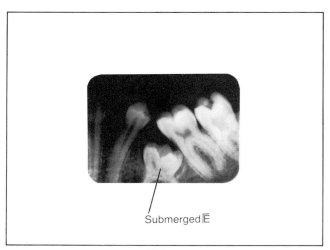

Submerged E̅

Figure 97. *Submerged E̅ in a girl aged 16 years. 4̅ and 6̅ have moved over the deciduous molar and the latter has become completely buried.*

that the vertical height of the crown of this tooth is less than that of the first permanent molar. The author feels that ankylosis of the deciduous tooth and growth of the alveolus supporting the first permanent molar is a more likely cause.

There are instances where the submerged tooth has almost disappeared in the young adult (Figure 97), and study of the vertical height here should settle the point.

The same submerged effect can occur if the first permanent molar becomes ankylosed.

References

Shafer, W. G., Hine, M. K. and Levy, B. M., *A Textbook of Oral Pathology,* Saunders, Philadelphia and London, 1958.

Stafne, E. C., *Oral Roentgenographic Diagnosis,* Saunders, Philadelphia and London, 1958.

3. Caries and Periodontal Disease

Caries

Extent of Lesions

It is an accepted fact, and can be shown histologically, that the caries process is more extensive than the radiographic radiolucency suggests. The typical enamel caries shadow seen in bitewing radiographs represents a lesion that has often reached into the dentine substance.

Depth of buccal, palatal, labial and lingual cavities cannot be accurately assessed radiographically. Often the caries shadow is superimposed over the pulp, but this only indicates the possibility of pulpal exposure, nothing more. The same can be said of interstitial caries shadows that are superimposed over the pulp.

The degree of radiolucency of a caries shadow is dependent on the amount of tooth tissue lying buccally, palatally, labially or lingually. Hence an interstitial cavity in a lower incisor will appear more radiolucent than a similar-sized cavity in a lower molar.

Oblique radiographic views of the crowns such as those produced using the bisected angle technique project a great thickness of enamel over the lesion, making interproximal enamel caries very difficult to see.

The Cervical Translucency

Radiolucent shadows are frequently seen on radiographs at the proximal edges of the cervical region of a tooth. These are not necessarily produced as a result of caries, but may be due to the difference in absorption by the enamel cap above and bone level beneath, compared to the area of dentine between (Figures 98 and 99).

Radiographic Views to Illustrate Caries

The Bitewing Radiograph

In the bitewing radiograph the patient bites on a card tab centred on the long axis of the film, so that the plane of the film is parallel to the long axis of the crowns of

Figure 98. *Diagrammatic representation of the cervical translucency. The enamel cap above and the bone level below cast opaque shadows. The area between, at the proximal part of the neck of the tooth, is radiolucent, and can easily be mistaken for radicular caries.*

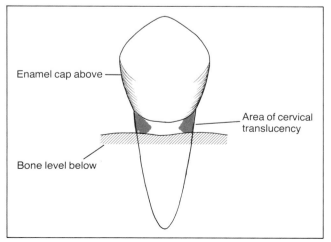

Figure 99. *Left bitewing radiograph illustrating the cervical translucency at the neck of $\overline{5}$. Unerupted $\overline{8}$ can also be seen on the radiograph of this 38-year-old man, in addition to interstitial caries.*

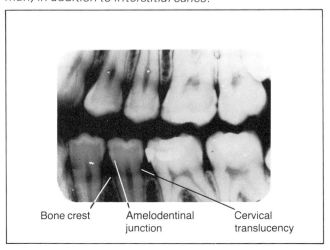

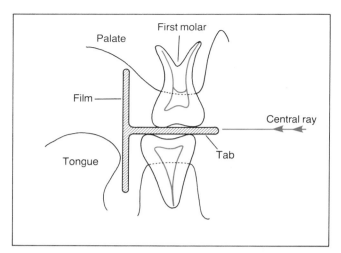

Figure 100. *Diagram of bitewing film in position showing plane of film parallel to long axis of molar teeth.*

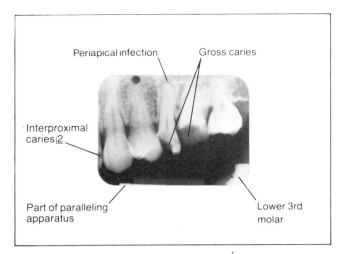

Figure 102. *Paralleling technique radiograph ⌊5-7 region. Similar vertical and horizontal projection to bitewing radiograph.*

upper and lower back teeth (Figure 100). The central ray is projected at right angles to the film.

The bitewing is the best projection to show interstitial caries from the distal aspect of the canines to the mesial aspect of the third molars—though it is not always possible to get all the contact points on the same film (Figure 101).

The Paralleling Technique Radiograph (The Long Cone Technique)

The paralleling technique radiograph provides an accurate view of the apices of the teeth covered, as well as

Figure 101. *Left bitewing film showing contact points from ⌊3d to ⌊7m. To include second molars distally and third molars mesially a second film would be required.*

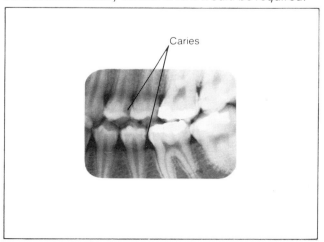

a similar projection to the bitewing for the crowns (Figure 102). However, they do not show both jaws on the same film, so at least four films are required to cover all of the posterior teeth.

Bisected Angle Technique Radiographs

Bisected angle technique radiographs are disappointing when used to illustrate caries. Because of the vertical angulation of the tube the x-rays pass through a considerable thickness of tooth tissue and early lesions may be obscured by this superimposition of tissue (Figure 103a and b).

Extraoral Radiographs

Extraoral radiographs should only be taken as a last resort to show caries. For young children and handicapped patients there may be no alternative. Oblique lateral and panoramic views of the jaws will show caries but are unreliable due to the superimposition of structures, and to poor definition resulting from the use of cassettes and intensifying screens.

The Appearance of Caries on Radiographs

Interproximal Enamel Caries

Interproximal enamel caries presents as a triangular radiolucency, usually at the contact point of the tooth with its neighbour, the base of the triangle being part of the enamel outline and the apex pointing towards the amelodentinal junction (Figure 104, ⌊5m 6m).

The decision has to be made as to whether or not the tooth should be filled at this stage, and the patient's age and predisposition to caries should be taken into account.

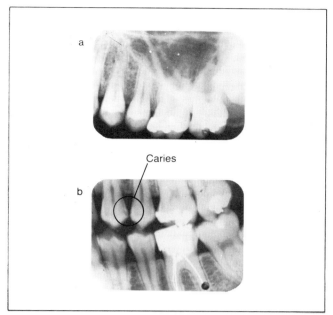

Caries

Figure 103 (a). *Bisected angle technique radiograph* $\underline{6}$ *region does not project any obvious caries. Bone levels are not well illustrated.* **(b)** *Bitewing of same region of same patient as (a) shows enamel caries* $\underline{5m}$ *and caries into dentine* $\underline{4d}$. *Bone levels are clearly illustrated in this view.*

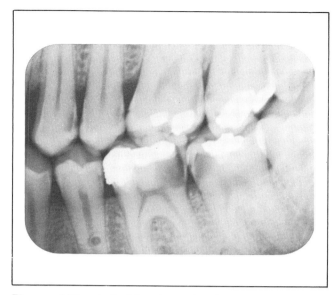

Figure 104. *Left bitewing showing: enamel caries* $\underline{5m6m}$; *caries to amelodentinal junction* $\overline{5d}$; *caries into dentine* $\underline{4d5d6d7m}$; *gross caries* $\overline{6d7m}$. *Bone levels are also clearly shown.*

Arrested Caries

Arrested caries may result at this point if the adjacent tooth is removed, the contact point becoming self-cleansing or readily accessible for the removal of debris (See Figure 113a).

There is a further type of arrested decay which is not often discussed. Following very extensive decay which has resulted in breaking away of the undermined cusps, a wide open cavity is left which is to a large extent self-cleansing or easily cleaned. The floor of this cavity tends to be heavily stained and hard, the tooth is still vital and there is no evident exposure of the pulp. The tooth may continue in this condition for many years without causing trouble (Figure 105). Generally one would expect to see the opacity of secondary dentine within the pulp chamber, and possibly the greater opacity of peritubular dentine beneath the cavity in the primary dentine.

Caries to the Amelodentinal Junction

When caries reaches the junction of enamel and dentine it spreads along the boundary as a thin radiolucent line (Figure 104, $\overline{5d}$). At this stage the enamel lesion may remain the same. It is generally considered advisable to fill such teeth, as the caries has undoubtedly invaded the dentine.

Caries into Dentine

By now a second radiolucent triangle can be seen on the radiograph, the base at the amelodentinal junction and the apex pointing towards the pulp (Figure 104, $\underline{4d5d}$).

Advanced Caries into Dentine

There is a continuing enlargement of the radiolucency as the caries extends further into dentine; by now there has

Figure 105. *Arrested decay* $\overline{7}$. *The occlusal cavity has become self-cleansing and the caries process has arrested.*

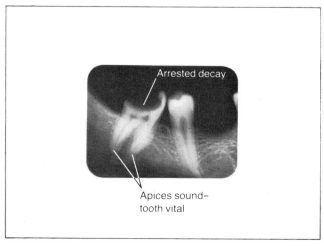

Arrested decay

Apices sound–
tooth vital

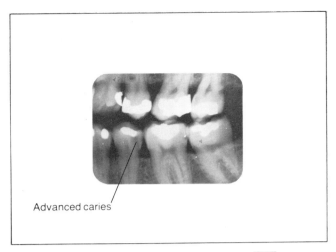

Advanced caries

Figure 106. *Advanced caries into dentine* $\lceil\overline{5d}$. *There is also caries* $\lfloor\overline{5d7m}$ *on this left bitewing.*

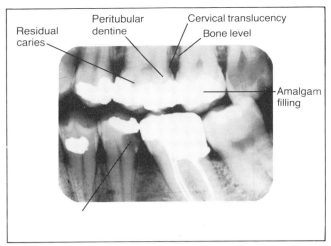

Residual caries | Peritubular dentine | Cervical translucency | Bone level | Amalgam filling

Figure 108. *Secondary caries can be seen in* $\lceil\overline{5d}$. *This has probably arisen through insufficient preparation at the cervical margin during cutting of the distal cavity. Residual caries can be seen occlusally under the filling in* $\lfloor\overline{6}$. *The cervical translucency is exaggerated by the amalgam filling and peritubular dentine, suggesting secondary caries distally in this tooth.*

usually been further undermining of the enamel (Figure 106, $\lceil\overline{5d}$).

In the healthy patient where the caries process has been fairly slow secondary dentine may well have been laid down in the pulp horn nearest to the decay, and the decrease of the pulpal radiolucency as a result of this will be evident on the radiograph (Figure 107). In rampant rapid caries the pulp will not always have had time to lay down this useful barrier.

Gross Caries — Likely Pulpal Exposure

Further decay results in the cusps being extensively undermined (Figure 104, $\lceil\overline{7m}$), and the carious lesion appearing superimposed on the pulp (Figure 104, $\lceil\overline{6d}$).

Clinical or histological investigation is necessary to confirm pulpal exposure, as the true extent of the lesion's depth cannot be gauged accurately from the radiographic appearance.

Secondary Caries

Inadequate extension for prevention at the cervical margin may result in fresh caries at this point (Figure 108). Badly contoured restorations with gaps and overhanging edges may also cause secondary caries to develop following food stagnation.

Figure 107. *Right bitewing showing secondary dentine has formed obliterating the distal pulp horn of* $\lceil\overline{6}$. *Secondary caries can be seen under the filling* $\overline{6do}\rceil$.

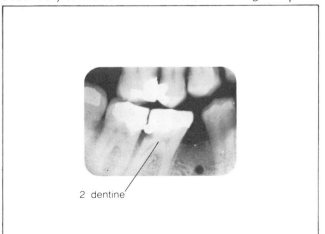

2 dentine

Figure 109. *Left bitewing illustrates residual caries under the amalgam filling* $\lceil\overline{6mo}$.

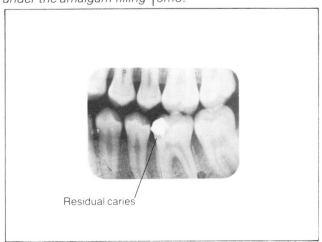

Residual caries

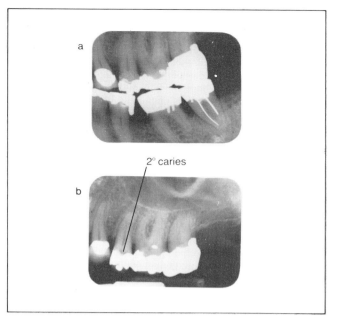

2° caries

Figure 110 (a). *Left bitewing with no obvious suggestion of caries under the filling in* ⌊5. **(b)** *Some 15° increase in the vertical angulation of the X-ray beam compared with (a). Caries can be seen under the filling in* ⌊5.

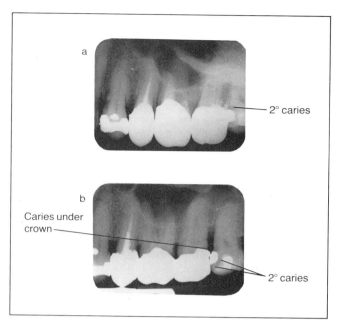

2° caries

Caries under crown

2° caries

Figure 111 (a). *Bisected angle technique radiograph does not suggest secondary caries distally under the crown in* ⌊7; *neither does it demonstrate bone levels well.* **(b)** *Same patient as in (a) using paralleling technique. Secondary caries can be seen under the crown* ⌊7 *distally, gross caries* ⌊8m, *and the bone levels are well illustrated.*

Residual Caries

Residual caries may be seen occlusally under fillings (Figure 108).

Inadequate preparation at the cervical margins leaving caries accessible to saliva will result in continuation of the caries process. Radiographs will reveal this state well in advance of clinical findings (Figure 109).

Secondary caries may or may not be seen on bitewing or paralleling technique radiographs depending on the contour of the existing restoration. In those cases where secondary caries cannot be shown with a horizontal beam it may become evident if some vertical angulation is used (Figure 110a and b). In those cases where secondary caries cannot be shown with a bisected angle technique radiograph it may be evident if the paralleling technique is employed (Figure 111a and b).

Confusion may arise between secondary or residual caries and the cervical translucency, particularly where a large interstitial filling reaches deeply down to the gingival margin. These cases are made even more difficult to interpret if peritubular dentine has been laid down deep to the filling. The contrast in opacity of the amalgam filling, the bone level and the peritubular dentine (which has an increased opacity to normal dentine), with respect to the translucency of the cervical dentine makes assessment difficult (Figure 108, ⌊6).

Occlusal Caries

Occlusal caries is seldom evident when confined to the enamel. The opacity of the latter obscures the early lesion in the majority of cases.

As soon as the process reaches the dentine an area of radiolucency can be seen, the outline of the deepest part being somewhat diffuse (Figure 112). The lesion may still appear small clinically when it has reached extensively into the dentine.

Figure 112. *Occlusal caries is well illustrated in* 76⌉. *Note the diffuse appearance of the lesions and the fact that they cannot be seen through the occlusal enamel. Unerupted* 8⌋ *and* 8⌉ *are evident.*

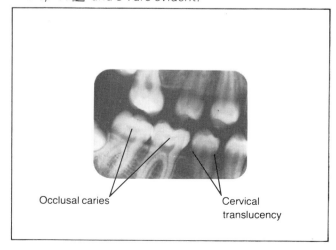

Occlusal caries

Cervical translucency

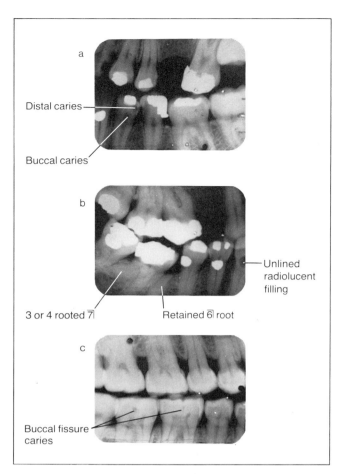

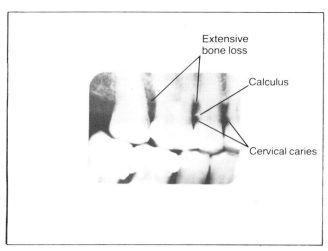

Figure 114. *Right bitewing exhibits marked bone loss with cervical caries 5d4d⌋. There is mesial caries in 7m⌋.*

Figure 113 (a). *Left bitewing illustrates buccal caries in ⌈4 (clinical examination would normally be necessary to say in which surface the cavity appears). Caries into dentine is also evident ⌈4do5mo. Enamel caries can be seen in ⌊5d and is probably arrested caries following removal of ⌊6. Radiolucency in ⌊3d is an empty cavity, the filling having been lost.* **(b)** *Right bitewing shows radiolucency of unlined silicate filling 3b⌉, confirmed clinically. It would be hard to tell from the radiograph alone whether the radiolucency was cavity or radiolucent filling material. Retained 6⌉ root can be seen, and 7⌉ appears to have at least three roots. The radiolucencies at the necks of*

$$\frac{7m6d}{7d}$$

are all highly suspect as possible caries. **(c)** *Buccal fissure caries can be seen in 76⌉ and there is little likelihood of this being in the lingual surfaces of the teeth. There is also bone loss and marked attrition of the teeth.*

Buccal, Palatal, Labial and Lingual Caries

These lesions (Figure 113a) can easily be confused with composite, plastic or silicate-filled cavities on radiographs, particularly when these are unlined (Figure 113b).

Buccal fissure caries can easily be seen in molars (Figure 113c).

Surface caries in posterior teeth may be obscured by an existing occlusal filling, so the radiograph is no substitute for a thorough clinical examination. The radiograph will not reveal whether the cavity is on the buccal or palatal surface of the tooth concerned.

On occasions the cavity may be mistaken for occlusal decay, but careful examination of the radiograph will usually reveal the sharp outline of the edge of the lesion in the enamel when buccally or palatally placed.

Erosion cavities buccally may give the appearance of caries on the radiograph and clinical examination is required in these cases.

Cervical, Cemental and Radicular Caries

These lesions present most frequently where there has been bone loss. They appear as radiolucent saucer-shaped depressions on the root interproximally (Figure 114). They have to be differentiated from the cervical translucency, and examination of all the teeth on the radiograph should help in the diagnosis. Clinical examination should settle the matter.

External resorption associated with periodontal disease can sometimes be mistaken for cervical caries, though sharp demarcation of the cavity is likely in the former, whereas the latter generally has a more diffuse outline.

In cases of bone loss cervical caries may arise at the neck of the tooth, invade the dentine and leave the enamel unaffected (Figure 115).

Caries in Children

The large pulps present in the deciduous dentition mean that caries should be dealt with as soon as possible.

The small films available for children (Figure 116) will cover the teeth from the deciduous canine to the first permanent molar. By the time the second permanent molar has erupted the child is able to tolerate the larger, standard size film.

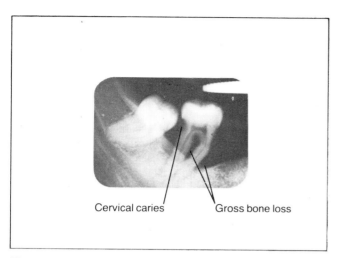

Cervical caries   Gross bone loss

Figure 115. *There is gross bone loss and cervical caries distally in* 7⌐*. The enamel does not appear to be involved in the carious process. The root of* 8⌐ *appears to be close to the inferior dental canal.*

Figure 116 demonstrates interstitial caries in

$$\frac{D \mid D}{D \mid DE}$$

and likely occlusal caries at the mesial end of the occlusal fissure E⌐ in an eight-year-old child.

Where very carious deciduous molars are near to being shed there is little point in their being filled; the likelihood of exposure of the pulp is high, with the attendant problems resulting. Good radiographs will clarify the situation.

Because of the large size of the pulp in the first dentition rapid caries is more likely to involve the pulp,

Figure 116. *Left and right small bitewing films of a child aged eight years. Caries can be seen in*

$$\frac{Dd \mid mDd}{dDm \mid DdEm}$$

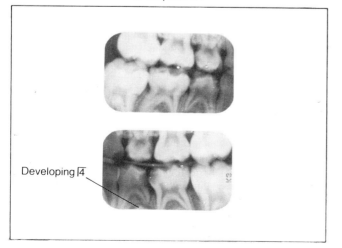

Developing ⌐4

even when the cavity appears average size, particularly in the case of the first deciduous molar.

Periodontal Disease

Good detail of bone condition and levels is required in periodontal assessment, so intraoral radiographs taken with a horizontal beam are indicated. In addition exposure times are best reduced by about one third to show the bone crest to full advantage. The exposure used for periapical assessment may well 'burn out' the crest of the bony ridge making assessment unreliable.

Radiographic Views to Show Periodontal Disease

Horizontal and Vertical Bitewing Radiographs

Horizontal and vertical bitewings are excellent projections to show bone crest levels of the posterior teeth (Figure 117a and b).

There are occasions when the vertical bitewing film is distorted due to the pressure from a low flat palate bending and pushing the film away from the maxillary teeth. In these cases the resultant bone levels will not be accurately depicted.

Bitewing films of the anterior teeth are generally unsatisfactory. The film is either bent by the tongue and palate, or is too far away from the teeth if a short cone is used. In addition the film plane cannot be placed parallel to the long axis of both upper and lower teeth at the same time.

The Paralleling Technique Periapical Radiograph

The paralleling technique periapical radiograph, using a long cone, results in accurate bone level projection, and this technique can be used for anterior as well as posterior teeth. With the aid of an appliance vertical and horizontal angles are determined and the central ray is projected at the centre of the film (Figure 117c).

The Bisected Angle Technique Radiograph

The bisected angle technique radiograph is very poor for demonstrating bone levels, and quite unsuitable for assessing bone loss at the bifurcations of teeth (Figure 117d). Buccal and palatal bone levels are projected at different levels on the film and a false impression is gained.

Extraoral Techniques

Orbiting panoramic projections. These can be very useful for a rapid general assessment of bone levels (Figure 118a). The vertical angle of the slit of rays is about 8° upwards throughout the exposure, and is therefore almost the same as a paralleling technique radiograph. From this valuable quick assessment the need for further films to show detail can be established, and then the requisite paralleling technique intraoral views taken.

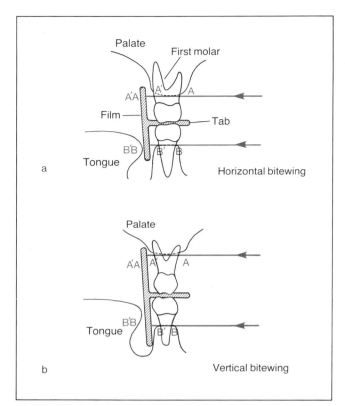

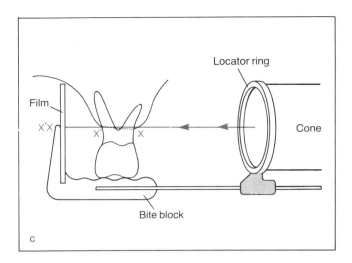

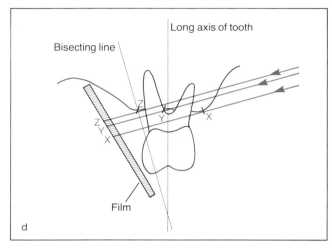

Figure 117 (a). *Diagram of horizontal bitewing in position. The card tab is fixed along the long axis of the film. The bone level from A to A' is projected accurately at AA' on the radiograph and B to B' at BB', as a horizontal beam is used.* **(b)** *Vertical bitewing in position. The card tab is fixed along the short axis of the film. Again bone level A to A' is projected accurately at AA' on the film and B to B' at BB'. When the patient has a low flat palate there may be bending of the top edge of the film resulting in possible inaccurate projection of the maxillary bone levels. Vertical bitewings are used when there has been extensive bone loss in the molar regions.* **(c)** *Paralleling technique, the central ray is projected at right angles to the long axis of the teeth and plane of the film. The X-ray machine cone butts onto the locator ring, setting correct vertical and horizontal angles and lining-up the central ray with the* middle of the film. The bone level X to X' is projected accurately at XX' on the film. **(d)** *The bisected angle technique. Bone levels X Y and Z are all projected at different levels on the radiograph although these points are all at the same level in the mouth. As a result accurate assessment of bone levels from the radiograph is not possible. Bone level X is projected on to the image of the crown. Level Z is projected at the same level as the apices of the buccal roots.*

Static panoramic views. These are taken with the x-ray tube in the patient's mouth and can be very useful in showing anterior bone levels (Figure 118b).

Radiographic Appearance of Periodontal Disease

Presence of Calculus

Calculus can be shown on radiographs particularly when a reduced exposure time is used. The opacity of the deposits can vary considerably, but even small amounts can be shown on bitewings (Figure 119). The gross deposits on lower anteriors are easily seen (Figure 120). Angulated views are not always satisfactory as the calculus may superimpose on the dentine and 'vanish'.

Localized Bone Loss

This may be caused by food packing in interstitial cavities and at the cervical margins, overhanging or

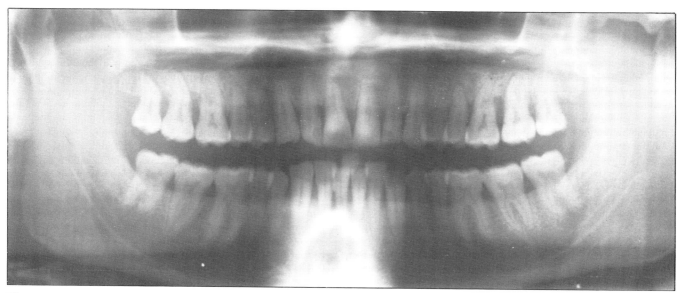

Figure 118 (a). *Panelipse (orbiting panoramic) radiograph illustrates bone levels well for general assessment. The vertical ray is angulated about 8° upwards throughout the whole 'pan'. Bone loss is greater in the maxilla here.* **(b)** *Panoral (static panoramic) radiograph of the mandible illustrates lower anterior region as far back as the first molars. The teeth are magnified considerably but the detail is good. The radiation dose is low.*

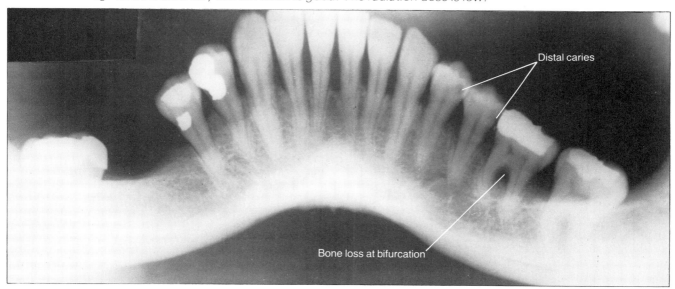

Figure 119. *Right bitewing radiograph showing calculus cervically on 76⌋. Bone levels are well shown.*

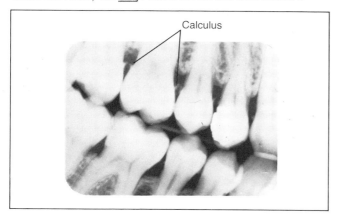

Figure 120. *Gross supragingival calculus with an opacity similar to dentine, can be seen on this radiograph. There is very extensive bone loss evident on this panoral radiograph and the bone crest is well seen in the original film.*

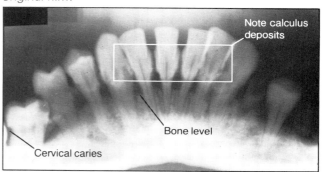

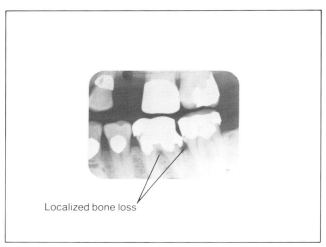

Localized bone loss

Figure 121. *Left bitewing showing localized bone loss probably related to food packing at the gingival margin ⌐6d. There is no proper contact point with ⌐7.*

deficient fillings, and badly fitting crowns and inlays. Figure 121 illustrates this condition on a bitewing radiograph. Food packing at the gingival margin and in the carious cavity ⌐6 distally has resulted in localized bone resorption with loss of the septal lamina and bone crest between ⌐67.

Chronic Periodontal Disease — Loss of Bone Crest

In chronic periodontal disease, which progresses if untreated, the tips of the bony crest are lost, and the later bone loss is horizontal and even (Figure 122a). It is a self-perpetuating condition and, unless treatment and instruction in oral hygiene are given, the bone loss continues (Figure 122b and c) until very little supporting bone is left. The eventual outcome is exfoliation of the teeth.

With arrest of the condition the lamina dura reforms

Figure 122 (a). *Horizontal bone loss illustrated on right periapical film, the crest lamina having been lost. The original film shows calculus deposits at the neck of 6⌐ distally. The patient is 34 years old. **(b)** Panelipse radiograph of patient aged 52, showing extensive horizontal bone loss, particularly in the lower jaw, with gross deposits of calculus. **(c)** Gross horizontal bone loss shown in periapical film. Teeth are loose clinically, though not spaced yet. The nutrient canals are shown well in this view.*

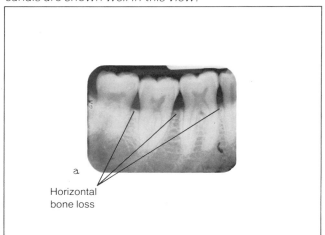

a

Horizontal bone loss

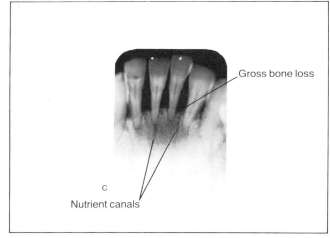

Gross bone loss

c

Nutrient canals

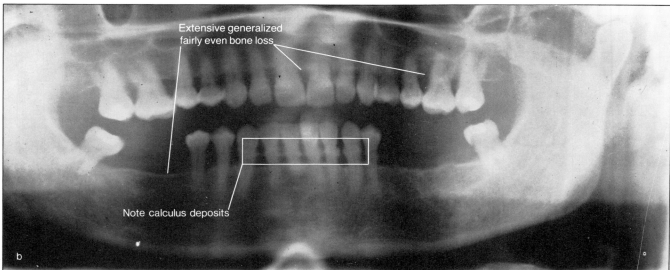

Extensive generalized fairly even bone loss

Note calculus deposits

b

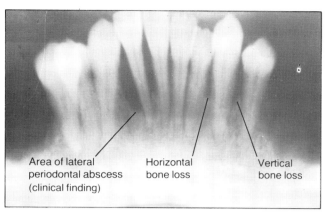

Figure 123. *Lower panoral view shows the appearance of chronic periodontal disease with irregular bone loss. There is marked vertical bone loss which is a feature of this disease. Lateral periodontal abscess was diagnosed clinically in 2| region, the tooth being tender and mobile. The patient is aged 38.*

across the ridge to be lost once more when the process becomes active again.

Chronic Periodontal Disease – Irregular Bone Loss

Vertical bone loss is the main feature (Figure 123) of this form of periodontal disease. It may be extensive and involve many teeth. Calculus deposits can generally be identified supra- and sub-gingivally, and tilting and separation of the teeth eventually take place. The septal crest lamina disappears early on, bone pockets form and the bone margins are ragged. Bone loss may be very uneven.

Periodontosis

Periodontosis is most often recognized as irregular bone loss around one or more teeth—frequently the first permanent molar and incisor regions—in adolescents or young adults with clean mouths (Figure 124). Apparently lack of an inflammatory process is a feature initially histologically, though in due course inflammation manifests itself.

There is no obvious cause for this condition, but bone loss can be very extensive indeed. In Figure 124 it is likely that |6 was extracted as a result of loosening rather than as a result of caries.

Widening of the Periodontal Membrane with Tooth Mobility

This is a progressively deteriorating condition. Lack of bony support results in loosening of the teeth and widening of the periodontal membrane, particularly towards the crest of the ridge (Figure 125).

Trauma to an isolated tooth may result in some subluxation giving the appearance of a widened periodontal membrane on the radiograph. This may not be the result of chronic periodontal disease, and the increase in thickness of the periodontal membrane will be even throughout its extent from apex to gingival margin.

Lateral Periodontal Abscess

The vertical bone loss seen in chronic periodontitis and late localized bone loss may give rise to lateral periodontal abscess. This condition is recognized clinically and can be confirmed with a radiograph (Figure 123). It can be mistaken for apical abscess clinically even though

Figure 124. *Panelipse radiograph showing extensive vertical bone loss in a woman aged 20 years. There is no suggestion of calculus deposition though there has been some generalized horizontal bone loss. |6 has been lost, probably as a result of loosening due to vertical bone loss, and periodontal abscess may have occurred during a period of lowered resistance of the patient, particularly if the bone loss had reached the bifurcation.*

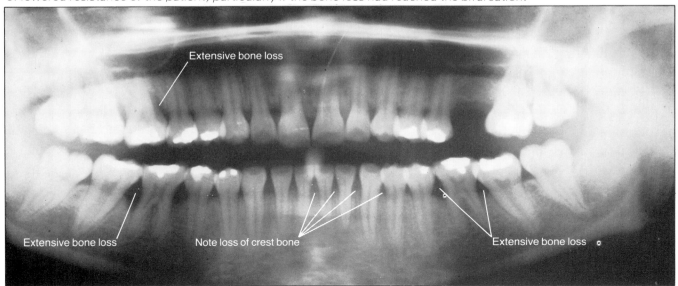

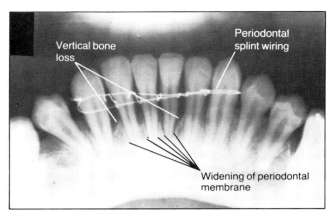

Figure 125. *Gross bone loss in the lower incisor region on a panoral radiograph of a man aged 21 years. Widening of the periodontal membrane can be seen and the teeth have been wired together as a temporary splinting arrangement because they were very mobile.*

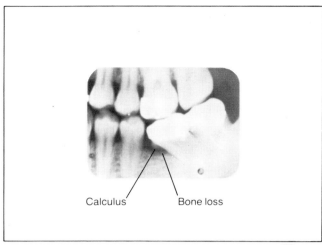

Figure 127. *Left bitewing shows early loss of ⌐6 with tilting forwards of ⌐7 and resorption of bone crest mesially to this tooth. A large deposit of calculus can be seen on the mesial aspect of tilted ⌐7. There has been generalized bone loss.*

there is neither caries nor filling in the tooth crown. The radiograph will show the vertical bone loss that has occurred, thus confirming the diagnosis of lateral periodontal abscess.

Changes of the Interdental Crest with Tilting of Teeth

In Figure 126 early loss of 6| has resulted in 7| tilting forwards with bone loss evident in front of the mesial aspect of this tooth. Calculus deposits can often be seen in such bad stagnation areas (Figure 127).

When a traumatic bite occurs as a result of the occlusion with the tooth above, widening of the periodontal membrane and movement of the tooth are to be expected. These events can be assessed from the radiographic appearance.

Changes of the Interdental Crest Following Vincent's Infection

In very bad cases of Vincent's infection the interdental papillae will be lost and the interdental bony crest will be destroyed. The radiographic appearance after healing will resemble early chronic periodontal disease, the lamina reforming in due course across the bone crest.

Bone Filling after New or Re-attachment Procedures

Radiographic assessment of the success of such procedures can only be made accurately with reproducible paralleling technique radiographs or bitewings.

Bisected angle technique radiographs are particularly misleading because of the variability in the angulation of tooth, the film and the x-ray beam.

Figure 126. *Right bitewing shows early loss of 6|, tilting mesially of 7| and vertical bone loss and pocket formation at this point.*

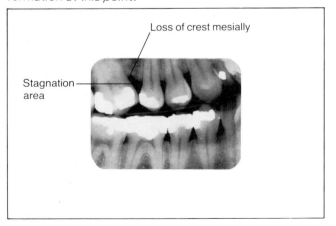

4. Results of Trauma

Dental practitioners are involved with trauma most of their lives, both creating it during operative procedures, and treating the results of it following accidents.

Radiographs are essential in most cases of trauma as a diagnostic aid to formulating a course of treatment, and for record purposes in case of possible litigation.

Trauma to Teeth

Conservation

Cavity preparation can be considered as one form of manipulative trauma, and excessive zeal may result in pulpitis, either transient or leading to death of the pulp.

Deep preparations frequently result in the production of secondary dentine in the related pulp horns and chamber, which is depicted as opaque obliteration of the radiolucent pulp shadow on the radiograph.

Abrasion

Excessive use of a toothbrush may result in abrasion cavities at the necks of teeth, and in severe cases there may be exposure of the pulp. This is usually when the pulp is unable to lay down secondary dentine fast enough to keep up with the destructive process. Care has to be taken that this condition is not mistaken for cervical caries when making radiographic assessment.

Attrition

This is a condition frequently found in the elderly patient and is regarded as a normal ageing process. The areas of wear are readily evident on radiographs as deficiencies of full coronal outline (Figure 128). Generally the pulp will recede from the crown, and the pulp canal will narrow within the root provided the process is relatively slow. A barrier of dentine will be laid down in advance of the worn areas.

A very heavy bite is sometimes the cause of attrition and it has been suggested that hypercementosis of the roots may occur in such cases.

Excessive attrition in the young patient can result in exposure of the pulps as the latter are unable to keep up with the destructive process and root treatment may be

Figure 128. *Upper panoral radiograph of a man aged 65 years showing marked attrition. There is calcification of the coronal pulps and narrowing of the radicular pulps. ⌊5 shows hypercementosis.*

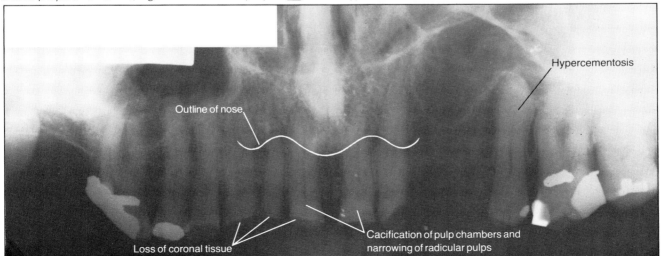

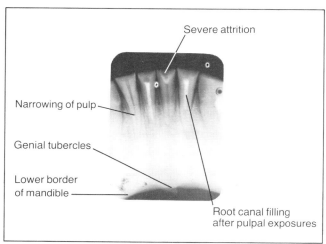

Figure 129. *Periapical radiograph of lower anterior region showing severe attrition in a young woman aged 23 years. Root treatment has been necessary as the pulps have been unable to keep pace with the wear process. The patient had a total of nine root fillings as a result of the attrition.*

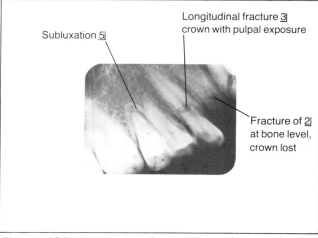

Figure 131. *Intraoral radiograph showing longitudinal fracture of crown and part of root of 3⏌ in a man aged 31 years. The pulp is obviously exposed. 5⏌ is subluxed.*

the treatment of choice. Figure 129 illustrates attrition in the lower anteriors of a patient aged 23 years. The upper incisors were also worn down to expose the pulps. In this particular case the attrition was due to bruxism, or grinding the teeth at night.

Coronal Fractures

Radiographically, coronal fractures can be divided into three groups:

1. Those involving enamel only.
2. Those involving dentine.
3. Those involving pulp.

Apart from minimal fractures of the incisal edge, fracture of the incisal angle is the most frequent coronal accident. Figure 130 shows horizontal fracture of the tip of 1⏌, and an angulated fracture of the incisal angle of ⏌1. In many cases it is not really possible to tell radiographically whether or not the pulp horns are exposed by the fracture, and clinical examination is necessary to be certain.

Figure 131 depicts a longitudinal fracture of the crown and part of the root of 3⏌. In this instance the pulp of the tooth was exposed. Longitudinal fractures tend to occur in posterior teeth that have been heavily filled, and where the cusps have been weakened and are no longer strong enough to take a heavy bite.

Figure 130. *Periapical radiograph of a boy aged eight years showing horizontal fracture of the tip of 1⏌ and fracture of the mesial incisal angle of ⏌1. There is no suggestion of radicular or alveolar fracture.*

Figure 132. *Periapical radiograph of a girl aged 12 years showing fracture of 1⏌1 roots with displacement of the fragments. There is marked elongation of the image.*

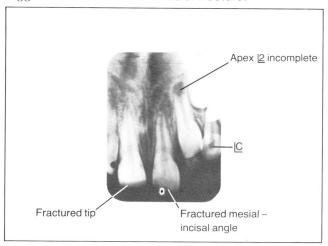

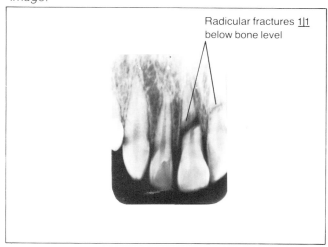

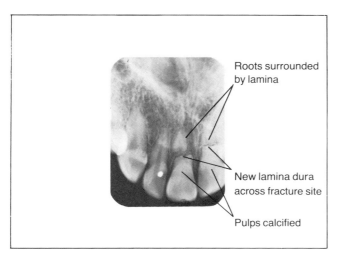

Roots surrounded by lamina

New lamina dura across fracture site

Pulps calcified

Figure 133. *Same patient as Figure 132 showing the condition of 1|1 three years later. There has been healing with the formation of a lamina across the fractured root ends. There is foreshortening of the image in this case.*

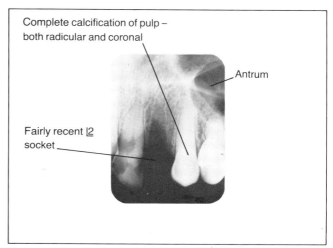

Complete calcification of pulp – both radicular and coronal

Antrum

Fairly recent |2 socket

Figure 135. *Periapical radiograph |23 region showing pulp of |3 completely calcified. The patient, aged 32 years, had a history of trauma to this region many years previously.*

Radicular Fractures

Transverse radicular fractures are the most common and may be at gum level or deep in bone. A direct blow is usually the cause. These fractures may be difficult to see radiographically if there has been no displacement of fragments, if there is just a crack, or if the fragments have overridden without lateral displacement. Figure 132 shows radicular fractures of 1|1 below bone with some displacement of the fragments. The teeth tightened up and three years later bone has been laid down between the fragments with a new lamina evident across the fractured root ends (Figure 133). There are no signs of any periapical changes, and the coronal pulps have calcified.

Figure 134. *Postoperative radiograph showing retained distal root of 6| below bone level. The mesial socket is empty. 8| has not yet erupted.*

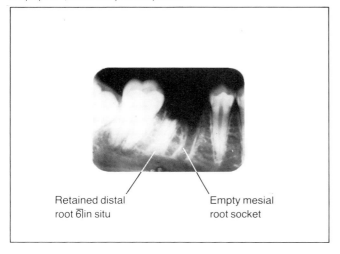

Retained distal root 6|in situ

Empty mesial root socket

Root fracture during extraction procedures (Figure 134) is an all too frequent occurrence, generally leaving the deep portion of root in situ. Radiographs at this stage are most useful for assessment as to whether urgent surgery is indicated for the removal of the remaining portion of root. In some instances it may be pertinent to leave well alone and allow the fragment to work its way out or remain enclosed in bone. Longitudinal fractures of roots (Figure 131) are unusual and generally confined to heavily filled premolar and molar teeth. Comminuted fractures of teeth are very unusual (Worth 1963).

Pulpal Response

A direct blow to a tooth may result in tooth death, internal and external resorption, or calcification.

Teeth of children with open apices are more likely to recover from trauma than those of adults which have closed apices. As so often Nature has made suitable arrangements for the accident-prone youngster! Figure 135 shows |3 with a completely calcified pulp. The patient, aged 32 when this radiograph was taken, had a previous history of trauma to this area when a youngster. The apex appears sound and the lamina is intact.

Figure 142 illustrates resorption of some bone and the root of 1| near the neck following direct trauma to the anterior teeth of this 15-year-old boy. |1 was reimplanted.

Dilaceration

Dilaceration is generally considered to occur as a direct result of trauma to a developing tooth; it is also possible that it may be a developmental anomaly. Figure 136 illustrates this condition, though in this case it is not

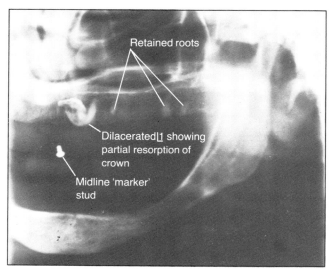

Figure 136. *Part of a Panorex radiograph showing dilacerated |1 with some coronal resorption. Retained roots are evident in the otherwise edentulous jaws, and the opaque 'stud' marks the midline.*

possible to say what was the cause as it was a casual finding on a prosthetic department's radiographic request querying the presence of retained roots. There appears to have been some resorption of the crown of |1 and the root may be overlying a retained root. Intraoral radiographs of the region are necessary to clarify the situation.

In cases of dilaceration seen on radiographs, careful assessment is required to avoid confusing the appearance with fracture, though the history will generally remove any doubt. Most cases of dilaceration, as is to be expected, occur in the upper incisor region, with the tips of the crowns pointing labially.

Figure 137. *Upper standard occlusal radiograph illustrating subluxation of 1|1 and fracture of 2|crown. Incisal angle fractures of 1|1 are not obvious on this foreshortened radiographic image.*

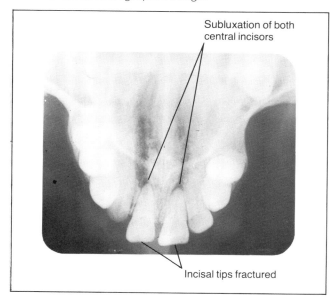

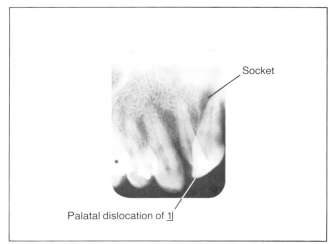

Figure 138. *Intraoral radiograph of a man aged 22 years showing palatal dislocation of 1|.*

Subluxation

Movement of a tooth in its socket by trauma may result in loosening. Figure 137 shows subluxation of 1|1; the periodontal membrane space at the apices is greatly widened, yet the teeth are still within their sockets. If these teeth are freed from the direct bite and splinted they may well tighten up and recover. Subluxation may be accompanied by coronal and/or radicular fracture, and radiographs should always be checked carefully for the additional possibilities.

The relationship of the tooth root to the lamina dura of the socket is an indication of the amount of displacement that has occurred. Teeth may be pushed into bone rather than loosened, and in such cases the radiolucent periodontal membrane shadow will be missing.

Dislocation

Dislocation is extreme displacement of the tooth, usually accompanied by fracture of the buccal or palatal/lingual alveolar plate of bone. Figure 138 shows dislocation of 1| in a man of 22 years. This intraoral radiograph shows the tooth to be markedly extruded from the socket, and indicates the displacement of the tooth palatally. Repositioning of the tooth in a young patient, and suitable splinting, may produce a favourable result.

Avulsion

Complete loss of the tooth from a socket may occur as the result of a blow (Figure 139). The radiographic appearance is similar to that of a socket following a normal extraction, as both events can occur with or without fracture of alveolar plates.

Reimplantation and Ankylosis

In cases of avulsion where the ejected tooth can be found and replaced and splinted under suitable con-

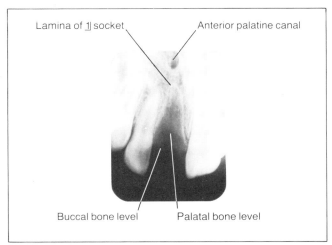

Figure 139. *Periapical radiograph of a boy aged 13 years showing empty socket of 1⌋ following avulsion of this tooth.*

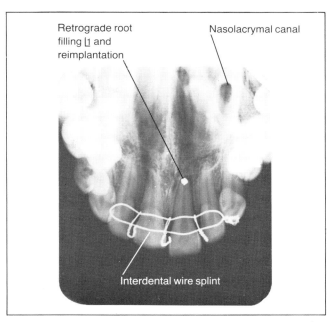

Figure 140. *Upper standard occlusal radiograph. ⌊1 has a retrograde amalgam seal and has been reimplanted. There is a wide radiolucent shadow between the root and the lamina dura of the socket. Interdental wiring splints the anteriors following trauma to 21⌋12.*

ditions, it may be possible for the replaced tooth to be retained for many years.

Figures 140, 141 and 142 illustrate such a case. ⌊1 had been forcibly ejected from its socket but was found and brought in by the patient. Following a retrograde amalgam seal the tooth was replaced in the socket and splinted with interdental wiring (Figure 140). At this stage there is a wide radiolucent band between the root and the lamina dura of the socket. There is no sign of bone change at the apex of ⌊1, and very little periodontal membrane shadow.

Figure 141 shows the condition 12 months later. There is bone loss at the neck of⌊1 and some resorption of the root at the distal aspect near the apex. The periodontal membrane radiolucency is absent, suggesting likely ankylosis. 1⌋ is showing definite periapical bone changes and there is some resorption of the root near the neck, and just possibly at the apex itself.

Nine months later (Figure 142) there has been further resorption of ⌊1 root, though the loss of supporting bone appears to have remained static. The tooth appears to be ankylosed. The apical area on 1⌋ seems to be static, but this interpretation can only be made with certainty after viewing serial radiographs of similar density and taken with similar angulations of tooth and film. Resorption of the root of 1⌋ at the neck is still evident, and there is the suggestion of slight bone involvement in this process.

The particular case discussed here is by no means the only possible form of reimplantation treatment, and operators have success without recourse to retrograde root canal filling. Whatever treatment is employed serial radiographs are essential for assessment purposes.

Root Canal Treatment Procedures

Perforations

Most of us have at some time or another perforated the apex of a tooth, either intentionally or inadvertently,

Figure 141. *Same patient as Figure 140, twelve months later. There has been bone loss at the crest of the ridge in ⌊1 region, some resorption at the apex of this tooth with possible ankylosis, and no sign of periodontal membrane shadow at the apex. In addition there is some bone change at the apex of 1⌋, and slight resorption at the apex and at the neck of the tooth.*

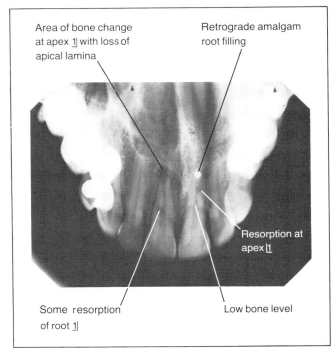

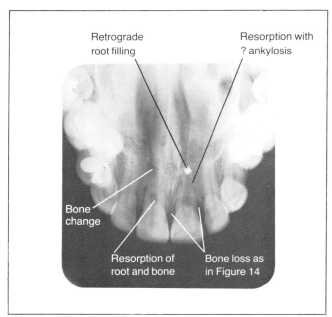

Retrograde
root filling

Resorption with
? ankylosis

Bone
change

Resorption of
root and bone

Bone loss as
in Figure 14

Figure 142. *Same patient as Figure 140, 21 months later, showing further resorption of* ⌊1 *root, certain ankylosis, but no obvious further bone loss at the alveolar crest. The area of bone change at the apex of* 1⌋ *is still evident, as is the resorption of root and adjacent bone near the neck of this tooth.*

Figure 143 (a). *Diagnostic wire reaching to the apex of* ⌈2. *The small radiolucent arc marking the radiograph is an artefact caused by bending the film across the end of a fingernail.* **(b)** *Root canal filling material has been forced through the apex of the same tooth illustrated in (a) into the periapical area of bone change.*

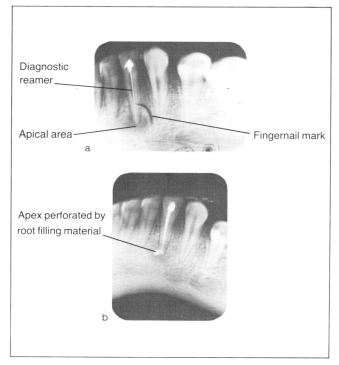

Diagnostic
reamer

Apical area

Fingernail mark

a

Apex perforated by
root filling material

b

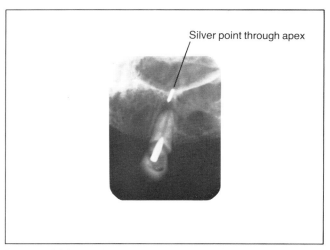

Silver point through apex

Figure 144. *Periapical radiograph of an upper canine with a silver point beyond the apex and related to the floor of the nose. There is a radiolucent area still evident at the apex of this tooth.*

during root canal procedures. Reaming through the apex may eventually result in root filling materials being pushed through the large apical opening into the surrounding tissues. Wide open apices of incisors create root-filling problems in children.

Figure 143a illustrates a diagnostic wire reaching to the apex of ⌈2. In Figure 143b root canal filling material has penetrated into the area of bone change in the same tooth. If this material is cement an apicectomy may be indicated. Figure 144 illustrates an upper canine with a silver point through the apex and beyond the area of bone change. A rather indifferent crown completes the picture! Lateral perforations of the root may arise during attempted removal of old root fillings or fractured posts, or when it becomes necessary to construct a post crown where the pulp has completely calcified. Without a postoperative radiograph lateral perforation

Figure 145. *Lateral perforation distally of* 2⌋ *root by a post. There is an associated area of bone change at the point of perforation and also at the apex of this tooth. Some resorption of the apex is evident.*

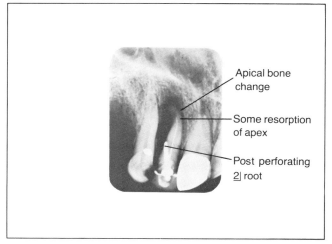

Apical bone
change

Some resorption
of apex

Post perforating
2⌋ root

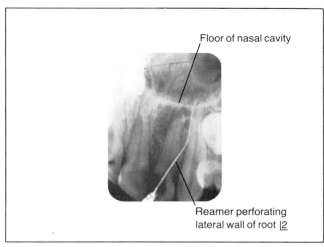

Figure 146. *Periapical radiograph of a man aged 22 years, showing a narrow reamer through a lateral perforation in ⌊2. There is an apical area of bone change on this tooth.*

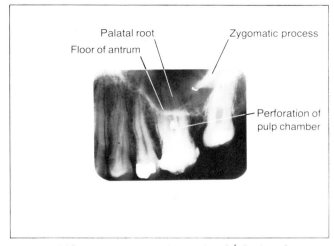

Figure 148. *Periapical radiograph of ⌊6 showing perforation of the floor of the pulp chamber and root filling material at the trifurcation.*

may pass unsuspected unless symptoms arise. The radiograph may show an area of radiolucency related to the perforation (Figure 145). This figure also shows some resorption of the apex 2⌋ and a bone change involving the apex.

It is only when a root canal instrument is in position that narrow lateral perforations can be demonstrated on a radiograph (Figure 146). The narrow channel in bone resulting from the instrument's penetration is seldom wide enough to be seen without the instrument in place.

If a large reamer has been involved in the perforation the canal made by this may be evident across the opaque root as a radiolucent band.

Lateral perforations can be repaired by 'patching' with amalgam (Figure 147), the procedure being similar to that for apicectomy and retrograde root filling.

Buccal or palatal/lingual perforations may not show on radiographs, and a tangential view of the suspect tooth should be taken if possible.

Perforations of the pulp chambers occur in some instances and these are nearly always between the roots at the bifurcations (Figure 148). Views at different angles may be required in the upper jaw in such cases, especially where the root fillings do not reach the apices.

Fractured Instruments

Spiral root fillers appear to fracture more frequently than any other root canal instruments, probably due to indifferent technique or old age of the instrument.

Figure 149 shows a fractured root canal filler lying at right angles to the long axis of the adjacent premolar

Figure 147. *Retrograde root filling and repair of lateral perforation in ⌊2 can be seen on this periapical radiograph. A further radiograph taken six months later would indicate the degree of healing that has occurred.*

Figure 149. *5⌋ appears to have two roots on this periapical radiograph, one of which is either very short, partly resorbed or apicectomized. A fractured piece of spiral root filler lies at right angles to the long axis of the roots. There is no history available for this case.*

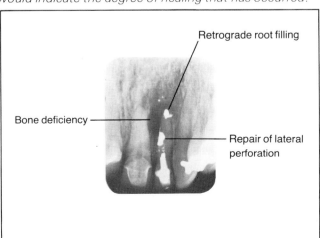

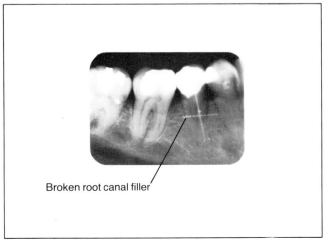

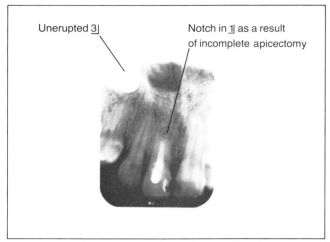

Unerupted 3|

Notch in 1| as a result of incomplete apicectomy

Figure 150. *Periapical radiograph of 21| region of a girl aged 17 years showing partial apicectomy of 1| that has healed completely with lamina formation within the notched apex.*

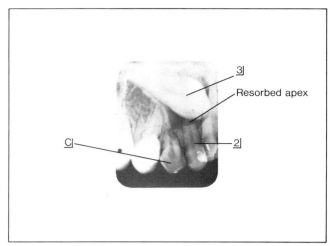

3|
Resorbed apex

C|
2|

Figure 152. *Periapical radiograph of 3| region showing marked resorption of 2| root apex by unerupted 3|, c| is retained also with some resorption, though whether or not this is related to the presence of 3| is debatable!*

tooth. The history of this accident is not known, but it is more usual for the broken fragment to remain in the root canal having got wedged near or through the apical foramen. This accident seldom causes ill effects.

Apicectomy

Being a surgical procedure apicectomy results in trauma to the root of the tooth and to the surrounding bone.

On occasions the patient is difficult or the field of vision is very limited. As a result the apices may not be completely removed. If the apical region is healthy the bone and lamina may reform in these 'partial' apicectomies, and Figure 150 illustrates such a case. Healing was uneventful in this instance.

Figure 151. *Periapical radiograph of 2| region of a woman aged 26 years showing complete apicectomy with healing. A new lamina has formed across the resection line, the apex is absent and bone has filled the space.*

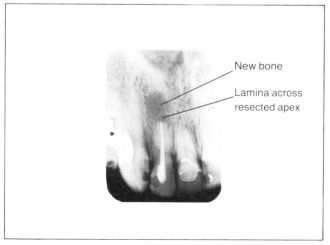

New bone

Lamina across resected apex

Following a successful apicectomy the lamina should reform across the severed root end after some time and appear continuous with the lamina of the rest of the socket (Figure 151). Often, as is seen in this radiograph, the root filling appears to be shorter than it should be. This is because either the resection line is angulated, or the x-ray beam and film are angulated to the tooth. Possibly both these factors contribute to the appearance in any one instance.

Resorption by Pressure

Heavy traction by orthodontic appliances, pressure from cysts, or unerupted and impacted teeth may cause resorption of the roots. In Figure 152 the pressure from unerupted 3| closely related to the lateral incisor has resulted in considerable resorption of the latter's roots. The same condition can be seen on lower second molars distally when mesioangular or horizontal lower third molars are hard against them.

Foreign Bodies

Foreign Bodies Produced by the Patient

Displaced Teeth and Roots

During surgery or as a result of an accident teeth may be displaced into other areas of the body, thereby becoming foreign bodies. Radiographs are essential for localization and record purposes, and two views are required, preferably at right angles, if possible.

Figure 153 is a lateral chest view illustrating the inhalation of a molar root into the right bronchus, confirmed by a posteroanterior view not illustrated. The boy concerned, aged 11 years, had multiple extractions followed by a dry cough and lassitude over a period of three weeks. He was admitted to hospital and the root

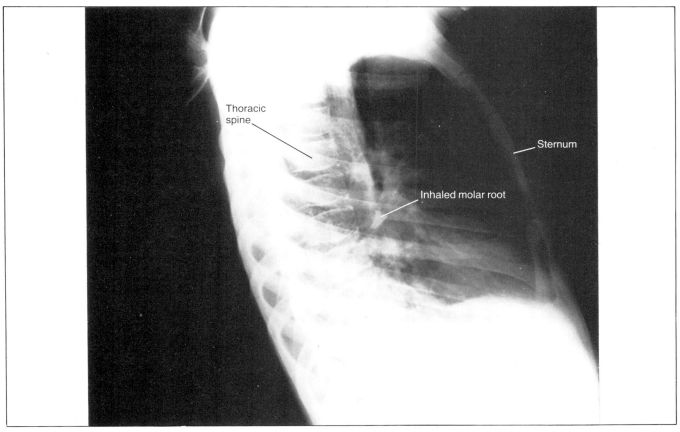

Figure 153. *Lateral chest radiograph showing inhaled molar root in the right bronchus. The 11-year-old boy had an uneventful recovery after removal of the root. A posteroanterior view is also necessary to localize the tooth.*

was removed under general anaesthetic. He was given penicillin and physiotherapy and a troublesome cough subsided three days after the operation, following which there were no further complications.

Roots are difficult to locate as the opacity normally provided by the enamel of the crown is missing. Figure 154 shows a swallowed upper third molar on its uneventful journey through the digestive tract. The opacity of the enamel makes the tooth easy to see.

Lower third molars may disappear under the soft tissue and into the lingual pouch, and if they cannot be located manually, radiographs in two planes may be necessary.

A relatively frequent occurrence is the pushing of a fractured premolar or molar root into the antrum, or under the latter's lining mucosa, during operative procedures. Carefully taken radiographs will indicate the position of the missing root. On occasions the root may have been displaced under the buccal or palatal mucosa and not into the sinus. Figure 155 illustrates a root of ⌊6 which appears to have penetrated the antrum, though it could be under the antral lining. The original periapical radiograph shows all three root sockets to be empty, and the occlusal view shows the root to be placed between the anterobuccal and palatal root sockets.

An oroantral fistula may result from attempted removal of roots from the first premolar to third molar

Figure 154. *Anteroposterior abdominal radiograph showing a molar on its way through the digestive tract, the enamel crown enabling the tooth to be located with relative ease.*

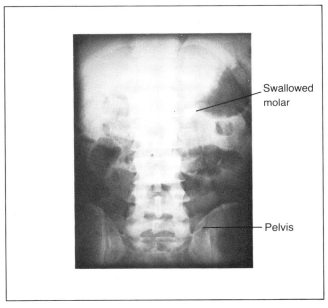

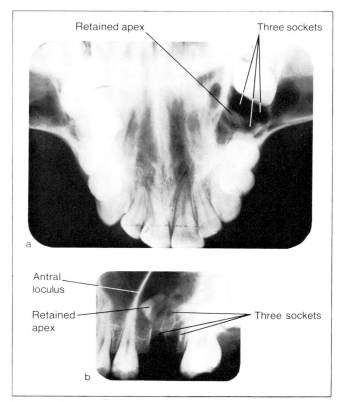

Figure 155. *Periapical and occlusal radiographs of a youth aged 17 years showing the root of ⌐6 in the antrum, or just possibly under the antral lining. The three empty root sockets can be seen on both radiographs, and the fact that the radiographs were taken in two planes enables the root to be located with accuracy.*

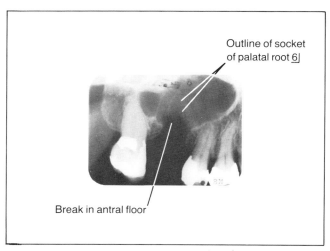

Figure 156. *Periapical radiograph of 6 ⌐ region showing deficiency of the antral floor indicating oroantral fistula. An accompanying occipitomental view (not shown) of this woman aged 42 years demonstrates an opaque right antrum.*

region. It is recognized radiographically as a deficiency of the antral floor (Figure 156), but often clinical examination will indicate the condition more readily than the radiograph. Fibrous tissue may replace the bony deficiency in which case there will be no clinical evidence of fistula though it will still be suggested radiographically.

Calculi

By lowering the radiographic exposure as much as one half most salivary calculi can be demonstrated. Figure 157 shows a calculus of the right duct to the submandibular gland. Views in two planes are essential as calculi can be mistaken for dense bone islands, odontomes, apical areas of sclerotic bone, and even unerupted teeth on lateral views. An occlusal radiograph shows that these salivary opacities lie outside the body of the mandible.

Phleboliths related to cavernous haemangioma (Figure 329), rhinoliths, and the calcification of glands can be demonstrated radiographically.

Implants

Figure 158 shows a metallic implant used to replace the left mandible after this section of the lower jaw had been removed for extensive ameloblastoma.

Figure 159 illustrates a metal plate used for immobilization purposes following fracture of the left mandible. The radiograph was taken some time after operation and there appears to be no reaction to the foreign body.

Figure 157. *Lower occlusal view showing a large molarform calculus of the right submandibular duct. The radiograph was taken as a result of finding a swelling in the floor of the mouth during routine dental treatment for this man in his 60s.*

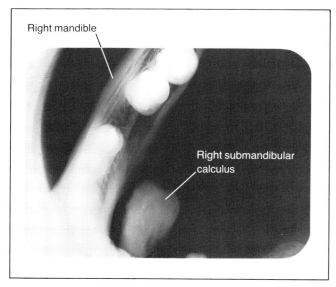

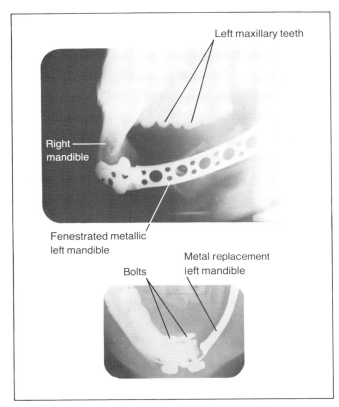

Left maxillary teeth

Right mandible

Fenestrated metallic left mandible

Metal replacement left mandible

Bolts

Figure 158. *Fenestrated metallic replacement of the left mandible seen on an oblique lateral radiograph of the mandible. The patient, aged 22 years, had excision of the left mandible for removal of an ameloblastoma. The lower occlusal radiograph shows the bolts holding the replacement left mandible in position.*

Figure 159. *Panelipse radiograph showing metal plate used to align and fix the left mandible some time previously for fracture of the body. Healing has been excellent and there is no suggestion of any foreign body reaction. Roots are evident in the maxilla and intraoral radiographs are advisable to show these in detail.*

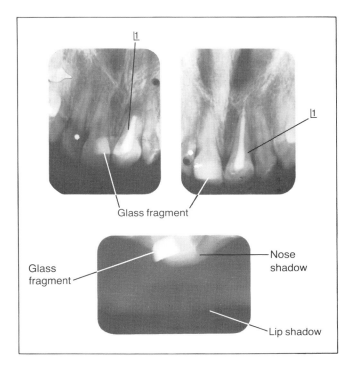

Glass fragment

Glass fragment

Nose shadow

Lip shadow

Figure 160. *Periapical radiographs show glass fragment in the upper incisor region. By parallax this is seen to be buccal to the arch of teeth, and the soft tissue view confirms that the fragment is in the upper lip. (For description of the case see the text.)*

Foreign Bodies Resulting from Accidents

Glass produces a lightly opaque image on radiographs, and the fragment indicated in Figure 160 was not noticed in the first radiographs. In point of fact both these teeth were root treated and later apicectomized in the mistaken belief that they were the cause of the patient's continual pain in this region!

Considering the two periapical radiographs in Figure 160 and using the parallax method (Chapter 2), it can be seen that the opaque fragment lies buccally to the arch of teeth. The soft tissue view confirms this.

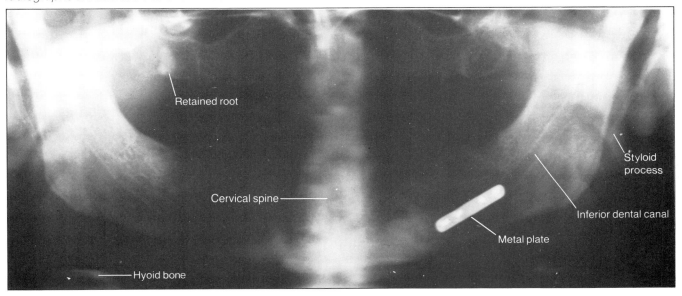

Retained root

Cervical spine

Hyoid bone

Styloid process

Inferior dental canal

Metal plate

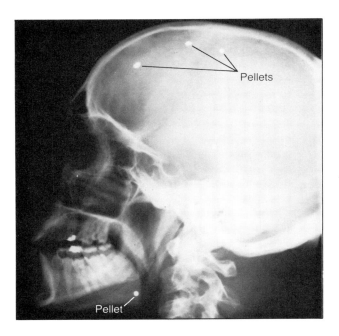

Figure 161. *Shotgun pellets seen on a lateral radiograph of the victim. A posteroanterior view would greatly assist in their localization.*

Figures 161, 162, 163 and 164 show pellets from a shotgun, an airgun pellet in the antrum, shrapnel, and an inlay in the piriform fossa, respectively. All these examples of foreign bodies require radiographs in another plane to show their exact position in the tissues.

Broken instruments occur from time to time and root canal instruments have already been discussed in this context. Figure 165 shows a broken bur head in $\lceil 8$ region occasioned during surgery for the removal of this impacted tooth. Suture needles sometimes fracture (Figure 166) possibly as a result of using tightly clenched forceps instead of needle holders.

Figure 162. *Airgun pellet in the antrum (or is it?). Another view in a different plane is indicated for exact localization of the pellet.*

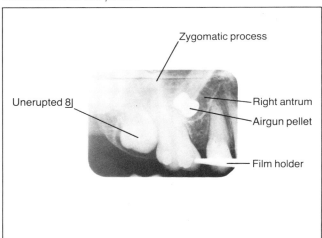

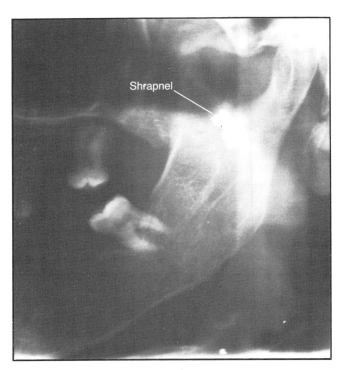

Figure 163. *Shrapnel related to the left ramus. A second view at right angles would show the depth of the foreign body below the skin surface.*

Prior to the manufacture of the disposable variety, fractures of hypodermic needles were not uncommon (Figure 167) and understandably the fracture generally took place at the point where the needle entered the hub.

Figure 164. *Lateral skull radiograph showing an inlay, possibly in the air tract. The inlay is in the piriform fossa, but a second view at right angles is necessary to confirm this anticipated position.*

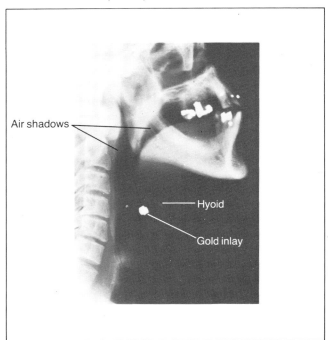

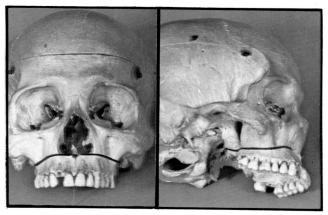

Plate 1, a and b. *Le Fort I fracture lines, frontal and lateral views.*

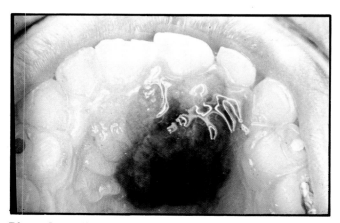

Plate 4. *Malignant melanoma of the maxilla.*

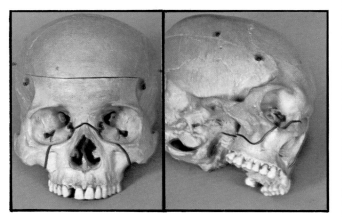

Plate 2, a and b. *Le Fort II fracture lines, frontal and lateral views.*

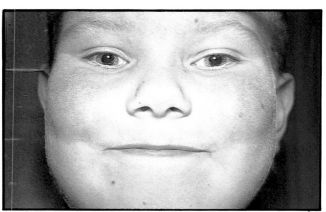

Plate 5. *Cherubism, or familial fibrous dysplasia. The subject does not show the true 'cherub' expression where the whites of the eyes are exposed, making the eyes appear constantly to look upwards.*

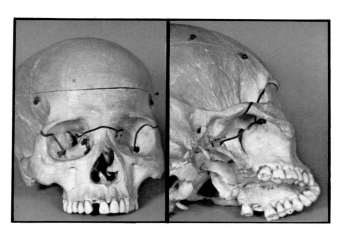

Plate 3, a and b. *Le Fort III fracture lines, frontal and lateral views.*

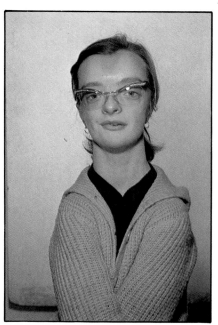

Plate 6. *Cleido cranial dysostosis in a 19 year old girl, showing frontal bossing and approximation of the shoulders.*

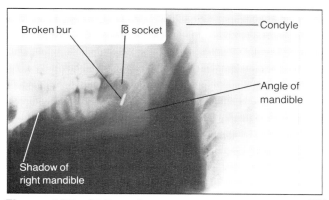

Figure 165. *Oblique lateral view of bur head in* |8 *region. A true lateral and posteroanterior view would be better, making localization more straightforward.*

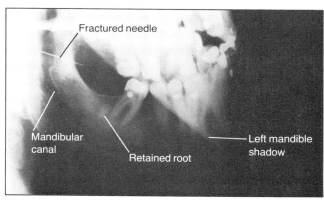

Figure 167. *Oblique lateral radiograph of the right mandible showing a fractured mandibular block needle. A posteroanterior and true lateral view would be a better combination, as they are at right angles to each other and would therefore make localization more straightforward.*

Fractures of the Jaws and Facial Skeleton

Radiographs should always be taken in cases of suspected fracture, even when the clinical diagnosis is obvious. In many instances more than one fracture is present, and failure to take adequate radiographic

views, apart from providing inadequate attention for the patient, may result in litigation. Detailed knowledge of the fracture site, extent and displacement are essential for the surgeon, and radiographs provide a great deal of this information.

Figure 166. *Periapical and occlusal radiographs showing position of a broken suture needle. A paralleling technique radiograph or a true lateral view would give a better idea of the level of the needle in the tissues rather than the bisected-angle technique radiograph seen here.*

Useful Radiographic Views

Bilateral fractures and compensating fractures of the opposite side can occur, and radiographic views should be taken with this in mind. Orbiting panoramic radiographs are of great help in assessing the mandible from condyle to condyle, but in addition some form of posteroanterior view is required.

The anterior regions of the mandible are poorly depicted in both panoramic and posteroanterior views, because the shadow of the cervical spine is projected across the incisor region. The intraoral lower occlusal radiograph is most useful for this area, both the true lower occlusal and the 45° lower anterior occlusal.

The middle third of the facial skeleton poses further problems as the bones of this region are very thin, and superimposition of structures in such views as the posteroanterior, occipitomental and true lateral make assessment of fractures very difficult. A number of radiographs taken at different angles are generally required.

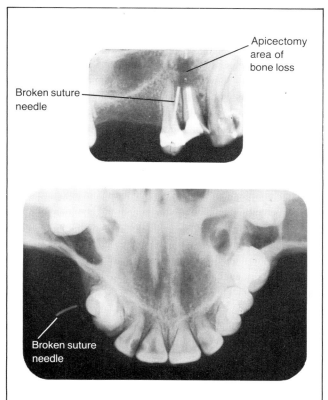

Visualizing the Fracture

Radiographs taken to illustrate fractures can be very disappointing, as the fracture lines may not be evident radiographically when the fracture is quite obvious clinically. This applies particularly to fractures of the facial complex.

The radiolucent line of break across the bone may be easy to see when the rays pass straight through the space between the fragments, but much less so when the rays are projected obliquely to the fracture line.

Displacement of the fracture ends may result in

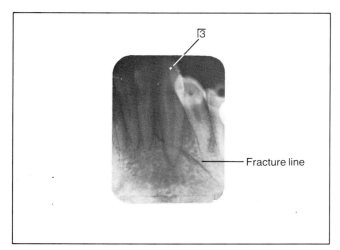

Figure 168. *Intraoral radiograph ⌐1-5 region of a boy aged 15 years showing alveolar fracture extending from ⌐2 region to below ⌐5. The patient had sustained a blow on the left side of the mandible. There was neither mobility nor displacement.*

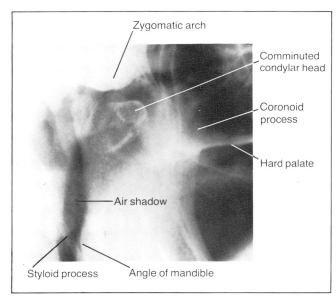

Figure 169. *Transpharyngeal view of the right condyle showing comminuted fracture of the head and displacement of the fragments. It is difficult to assess the number and lateral position of the fragments, though they have moved downwards and forwards.*

widening of the radiolucent fracture line, or a step in the bony contour where lateral shift of the bone fragments has taken place. Where lateral displacement has occurred, over-riding of the fragments may take place, so that radiographically there may be no step in one plane. This will make the diagnosis of fracture uncertain, hence views in a different plane are always advantageous. Fracture of the condylar neck often appears with overlapping on the lateral view.

'Greenstick' fractures of the jaws may occur in the younger patient, frequently involving the neck of the condyle, the bone wrinkling rather than fracturing across. Radiographs show the outline shape change when taken in the correct plane. The deformity may be very slight and is then easily missed on the radiographs.

A fracture of the mandible involving both buccal and lingual plates may be projected as two separate radiolucent lines, and these should not be taken as representing a comminuted fracture. The lines will tend to meet at their extremities, showing that they represent a single fracture through bone. This appearance is often evident on radiographs of fractures of the mandible.

An error of diagnosis may occur when viewing oblique and true lateral radiographs. A radiolucent line caused by the air space between the back of the tongue and the lower surface of the soft palate may suggest a fracture line if the two structures are almost touching. The fact that the air shadow continues beyond the lower border of the mandible should be sufficient evidence to prevent the misdiagnosis of fracture.

Alignment and Union

Pathological fractures may occur in lesions of the jaws, for example cysts, osteomyelitis or tumours. Surgeons sometimes find it advantageous to have splints made in advance of operations on such large lesions, in case of fracture during the operation.

Deliberate surgical fractures are made in repositioning procedures of the jaws for cosmetic purposes, for example saggital split operations on the mandible.

Radiographs are required after repositioning and fixation of the bone fragments to make certain that alignment is adequate in all planes. This is important as the alignment may look excellent on an anteroposterior view, yet poor on a lateral view, and vice versa.

Clinical union will have occurred well before the fracture line has disappeared from the radiograph. Fibrous union, or non-union, may occur in undetected fractures or fractures that have been inadequately immobilized. Sequestration of fragments may occur where there is an inadequate blood supply to the fragment, or when infection of the area occurs.

Fractures of the Mandible

For radiological assessment, fractures of the mandible can be subdivided into:

1. Alveolar.
2. Condylar.
3. Coronoid.
4. Ramus.
5. Angle.
6. Body.
7. Symphysis.

These fractures may be complete or incomplete, simple, compound, comminuted or 'greenstick'.

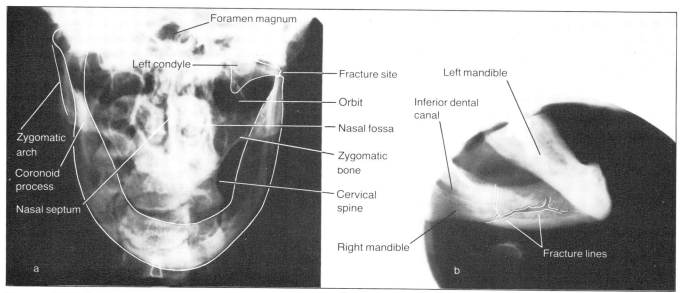

Figure 170 (a). *Posteroanterior view of the condyle of a man aged 49 years showing fracture of the neck of the left condyle and displacement of the head medially. There is no evidence of fracture of the right condyle. The outlines of the cervical vertebrae cause confusion, suggesting additional fractures in the anterior part of the mandible.* **(b)** *Oblique lateral view of the same patient showing fractures of the body of the right mandible in $\overline{76}\backslash$ region from lower to upper border, and also running transversely forwards towards the mental foramen region.*

Alveolar Fractures

Alveolar fractures can be sustained as the result of a blow. Figure 168 shows alveolar fracture of $\overline{2\text{-}5}$ region in a boy aged 15 years following a blow to the face. There was no mobility of the region, neither was there any sign of fracture apart from swelling.

Extraction procedures may cause alveolar fractures of the mandible. The typical socket expansion made with forceps prior to the removal of a tooth is seldom evident on intraoral views of the mandible, as it is often a type of 'greenstick' fracture. Generally speaking, fracture of the buccal or lingual plate during the extraction of a lower tooth will result in the bone being removed with the tooth. Sometimes patients return following extractions with discomfort in the area of the socket, and a piece of buccal or lingual bone, or the septum, is found to be mobile and separating from the rest of the mandible. An intraoral radiograph will generally show the extent of the fracture.

Condylar Fractures

Fractures of the condyle can be divided broadly into two groups: intracapsular and extracapsular.

Intracapsular Fractures

Intracapsular fractures of the condyle involve the articular surface and are difficult to show well on radiographs. Transpharyngeal (Figure 169), occipitomental, posteroanterior and tomographic views are best. Crushing of the articular surface is sometimes seen in children, and the two main complications are ankylosis and possible interference of the growth centre; the first

resulting in interference with the range of movement of the damaged condyle, and the latter possibly resulting in an uneven growth pattern between the left and right sides of the mandible.

Extracapsular Fractures

Extracapsular fractures of the condyle are common. They are most commonly unilateral, often presenting as a compensating fracture associated with a body fracture of the opposite side (Figures 170, a and b), or bilateral (Figure 171), usually the result of direct impact to the

Figure 171. *Posteroanterior view showing bilateral fractures of the condyles of a man aged 30 years. The condylar heads have displaced forwards, medially and downwards on to the articular eminence.*

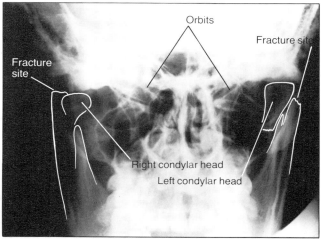

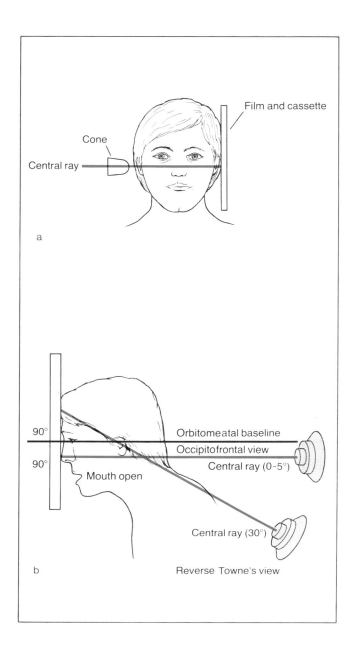

Figure 172. *Radiographic positioning for:* **(a)** *Transpharyngeal projection with mouth open. The cassette is held close against the side of the face covering the ear and with the head erect. The tube is centred one inch in front of the ear, through the sigmoid notch, and below the zygomatic arch on the side opposite to that required. The central ray is projected perpendicular to the saggital plane. This view shows the ramus, condyles if the mouth is open, and the angle of the jaw. The posterior aspect of the maxilla is also depicted.* **(b1)** *The occipitofrontal posteroanterior with or without mouth open. This is a good view for the ramus and middle and posterior part of the body of the mandible.* **(b2)** *The reversed Towne's posteroanterior with mouth open. This is an excellent view to show condylar heads and necks and is the posteroanterior projection of choice for illustrating fracture of these structures.*

chin. The amount of displacement of the condylar head is very variable, though generally it is found to have been pulled downwards, forwards and inwards. To demonstrate these fractures, oblique lateral views can be added to those used to show intracapsular fractures.

It is sometimes difficult to recognize a condylar fracture on one type of radiographic view, so it is very important to have views taken in different planes. Over-riding of the fragments, particularly on lateral views, can cause confusion, and an additional posteroanterior radiograph is essential to show medial or lateral displacement.

Figure 172 shows the positioning for the transpharyngeal, the posteroanterior occipitofrontal, and the posteroanterior reverse Towne's radiographic views. The mouth is opened in an attempt to move the condylar head downwards and forwards on to the articular

Figure 173 (a). *Transpharyngeal radiograph showing crack fracture extending from the sigmoid notch to the lower part of the back of the right ramus, a very low condylar fracture. The fracture line is easily lost in the overlying air space shadow.* **(b)** *Posteroanterior view of the same patient shows angulation of the right side of the mandible near the sigmoid notch, suggesting 'greenstick' fracture, with slight displacement laterally of the condylar head. The patient is aged 17½ years. There is also a fracture of ⌐3 region not seen on these radiographs.*

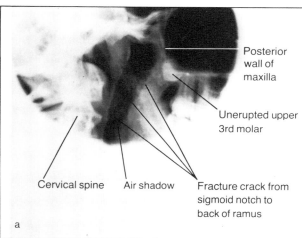

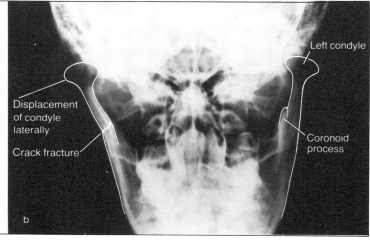

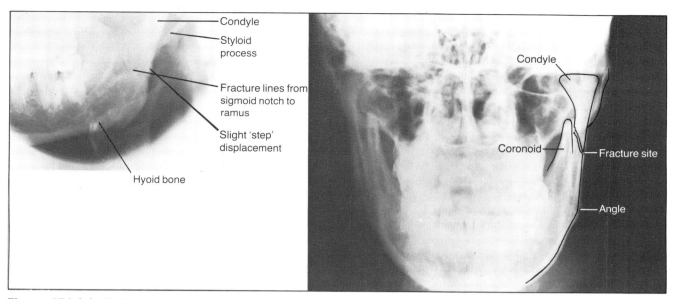

Figure 174 (a). *Oblique lateral view of patient aged 34 years showing fracture lines from the sigmoid notch to the posterior aspect of the left ramus.* **(b)** *Posteroanterior view of the same patient illustrates definite fracture line with little displacement evident. The right condyle does not show any sign of fracture.*

eminence and out of the shadow of the glenoid fossa. The reverse Towne's is the posteroanterior projection of choice to show the condylar heads and necks, and the posteroanterior occipitofrontal is the projection of choice for fractures of the ramus and body of the mandible (as well as lateral views).

Low condylar fractures may present as a crack starting in the glenoid fossa and running downwards and backwards on the transpharyngeal (Figure 173) or oblique lateral radiograph. The posteroanterior view shown in Figure 173 illustrates lateral 'bending', suggestive of 'greenstick' fracture, and the true diagnosis requires assessment of both radiographs. Figure 174a

and b shows the same type of fracture, with more obvious displacement of the fragments.

Suspected fracture of the condyle is not adequately demonstrated in Figure 175a, as no step can be seen in the outline of the condylar head shadows, but the left transpharyngeal view (Figure 175b), shows a high condylar fracture with an obvious step in the head contour, the head being displaced forwards.

Figure 176 reveals a 'greenstick' fracture towards the base of the right condyle, with a trace of outward angulation, but no displacement of the fragment ends, which remain in good contact. The oblique lateral view (not shown) indicates no fracture present.

Figure 175 (a). *Posteroanterior view of condyles of a man aged 32 years with no obvious sign of fracture or displacement.* **(b)** *Transpharyngeal view of left condyle showing high fracture and forward tilting of the head. If Figure 175a is reviewed, this malposition becomes evident.*

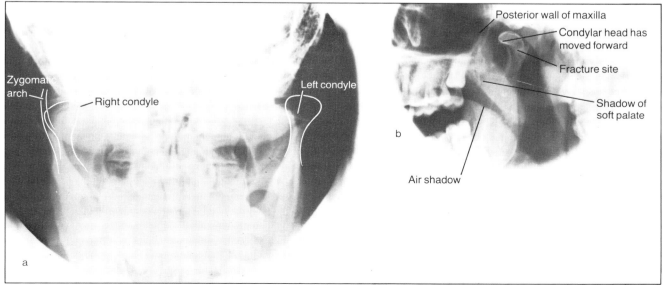

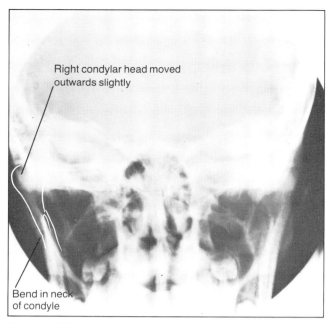

Figure 176. *Posteroanterior radiograph of a child aged 13 years showing 'greenstick' fracture of the neck of the right condyle. The head has moved outwards slightly. There is no fracture line evident in either this view or the transpharyngeal view (not shown).*

A very rare fracture of the glenoid fossa occurs when the condylar head is forced through the glenoid fossa into the midcranial fossa (Figure 177). In this instance the patient was unable to move the lower jaw at all, and condylectomy was necessary to regain active movement. Healing was uneventful.

Fractures of the Coronoid Process

Fracture of the coronoid process is rare, and it is difficult to diagnose on clinical examination. Oblique

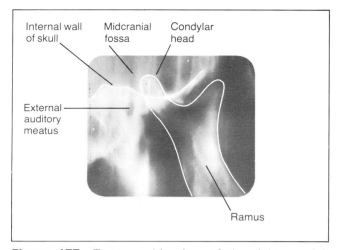

Figure 177. *Tomographic view of the right condyle showing the head forced through the glenoid fossa into the midcranial fossa. Condylectomy was necessary before the patient could move his lower jaw.*

lateral views will sometimes show the fracture (Figure 178a), though often the radio-opaque shadow of the soft palate covers this region on this type of radiograph. Posteroanterior (Figure 178b) and occipitomental views will show the fracture lines and displacement better. Pull of the fibres of the temporal muscle tends to separate the two fragments.

Fractures of the Ramus

Fractures of the ramus are relatively rare and can be seen on panoramic, posteroanterior and oblique lateral views. Figure 179 is an oblique lateral radiograph showing crack fracture of the lower aspect of the ramus extending backwards from 8|. The two radiolucent lines seen on the radiographs in Figures 179 and 180a depict

Figure 178 (a). *Oblique lateral view of a man aged 24 years showing transverse fracture of the right coronoid process —though not very clearly.* (b) *Posteroanterior radiographic view of the same patient showing fracture of the coronoid process, with little displacement, associated with fracture of the right condyle. In addition there was a body fracture in |2 region evident on an oblique lateral view of the left mandible (not shown).*

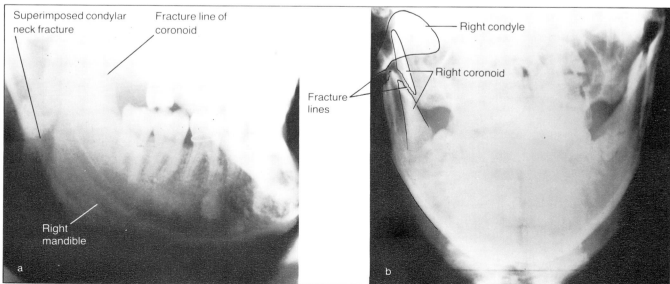

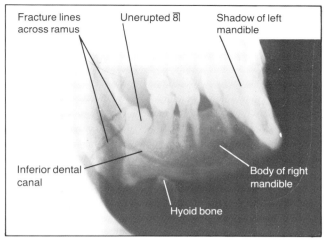

Figure 179. *Oblique lateral radiographic view of the right mandible showing crack fracture with little displacement through the distal edge of $\overline{8|}$ crypt and across the lower part of the ramus. $\overline{8|}$ is unerupted in this man aged 42 years.*

fracture of the buccal and lingual plates of bone, as can be seen from studying the posteroanterior view of Figure 180b. These double lines should not be confused with comminuted fractures (see Figure 184a and b).

There is seldom much displacement in these cases as the masseter holds the fragments together unless there has been extreme violence.

Fractures of the Angle

Fractures of the angle may be caused by attempted removal of buried third molars, and will usually result in a diagonal fracture line through the lower third molar region downwards and backwards to the outside angle. This is an unfavourable fracture line, and the anterior edge of the posterior fragment will tend to rotate upwards as a result of muscular action (Figure 181a and b). If a molar is retained in this posterior fragment and is in occlusion with its opposite number, alignment is

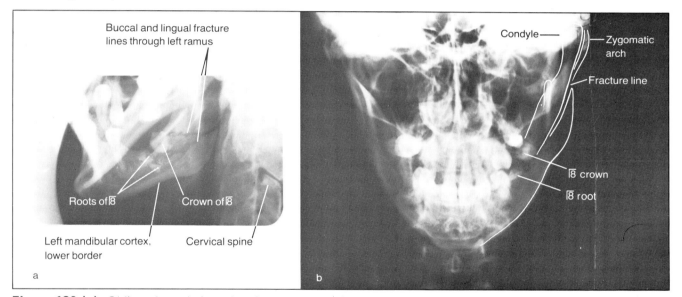

Figure 180 (a). *Oblique lateral view showing transverse fracture through the left ramus of a woman aged 31 years, involving $\overline{|8}$ with separation of the crown and roots. The two fracture lines that can be seen crossing the ramus are the buccal and lingual plate fracture lines and do not represent a comminuted fracture.* (b) *The angulated fracture line from buccal to lingual plate can be seen on this posteroanterior radiographic view and explains the two lines seen in Figures 179 and 180a.*

Figure 181 (a). *Oblique lateral view of the left mandible of a man aged 44 years showing fracture through the socket following attempted extraction of $\overline{|8}$ four days previously with some displacement. The fracture line is unfavourable.* (b) *Removal of $\overline{|8}$ from the fracture line and interdental wires to immobilize the jaws can be seen in the same patient. There is still some displacement of the fragments.*

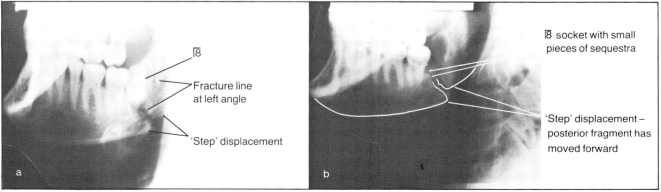

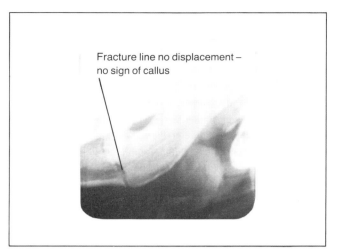

Figure 182. *Oblique lateral radiograph of a man aged 32 years showing fracture line through ⌐8 socket downwards to slightly in front of the left angle. Interdental wiring is present and the posterior fragment is fixed by the molar still present which prevents upwards rotation. There was clinical union at this stage, though no callus can be seen, and the fixation was removed following the taking of this radiograph.*

more straightforward, as the tooth will prevent rotation of the fragment (Figure 182), even though the fracture line is unfavourable.

Fractures of the Body

Figure 183, an orbiting panoramic view (Panelipse), shows fracture of the mandible in $\overline{5|8}$ regions with little displacement. The mylohyoid is attached on either side of the fracture line and will tend to draw the fragments together. The two radiolucent lines seen in the fracture

Figure 183. *Panelipse radiograph showing bilateral fracture of the mandible $\overline{5|8}$ regions. The two fracture lines in ⌐8 region are the buccal and lingual plate fractures. The left earring casts a dense opacity over the right coronoid process, making assessment of fracture or the right coronoid impossible in this view. $\overline{5|}$ in the fracture line has periapical infection, as do $\overline{6|7}$.*

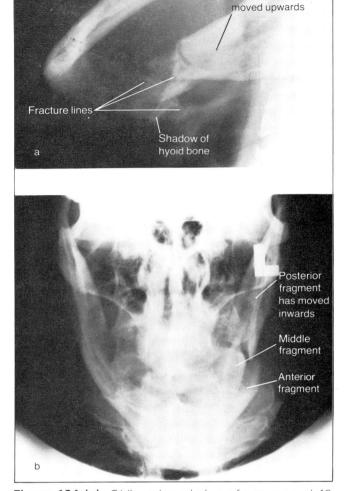

Figure 184 (a). *Oblique lateral view of a man aged 49 years showing comminuted fracture of the left mandible with marked upward displacement and over-riding of the posterior fragments. The mental foramen can be seen.* (b) *Posteroanterior view of the same patient showing fracture of the left mandible and medial displacement of the posterior fragments. There is no suggestion of condylar fracture.*

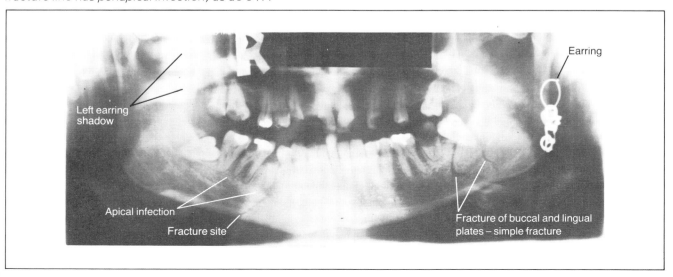

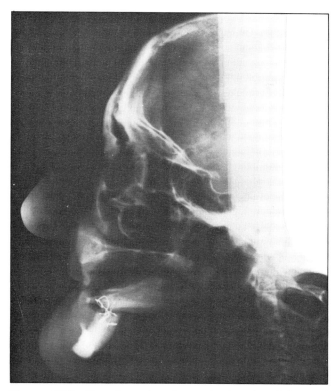

Figure 185. *True lateral radiograph showing failure of bilateral body fracture of the mandible to unite. The patient was old and had been immobilized for some time. Muscles attached to the genial tubercles have pulled the fragment downwards and backwards.*

of the left side are the fracture lines of buccal and lingual plates.

Body fractures may be comminuted, and in the particular case shown in Figure 184a and b, an edentulous mandible, there has been marked displacement.

Bilateral body fractures of the edentulous mandible may fail to unite due to the age and debility of the patient. Generally it is not possible radiographically to show callus formation at the fracture site (Worth 1963), thereby making it difficult to assess the stage of repair.

Figure 185 illustrates failure of union of bilateral fracture of the edentulous mandible where the muscles attached to the genial tubercles have pulled the anterior bone fragment downwards and backwards. Repositioning and the insertion of metal plates were required in this instance.

Fracture of the mandible in the canine region can be shown well, both on well-rotated oblique lateral views and on lower occlusal views (Figure 186a and b).

Fractures at the Symphysis

Fractures occurring just to one side of the genial tubercles (Figure 187) will often show marked displacement on the occlusal radiograph as the genial muscles will pull the larger fragment, which includes the tubercles, inwards.

Figure 188 shows an oblique fracture across the symphysis with little displacement.

Fractures of the Maxilla and Facial Skeleton

Fractures involving the maxilla, zygomatic complex and nasal complex may be difficult to show radiographically, and a negative finding on occipitomental radiographs is not necessarily a true indication of the situation. Very careful assessment is required and several views are necessary. Difficulty in interpretation is caused because the bones are very thin, and there may be overlying structures to confuse the assessor.

Figure 186 (a). *Well-rotated oblique lateral view of a man aged 34 years showing body fracture of the left side of the mandible with some displacement. The shadow of the hyoid bone crosses the body of the mandible in ⌐6 region. There was also a fracture of the base of the left condyle, but it does not show in this view.* **(b)** *An obliquely placed lower occlusal film of the same patient, showing the fracture in ⌐3 region extending towards the genial tubercles.*

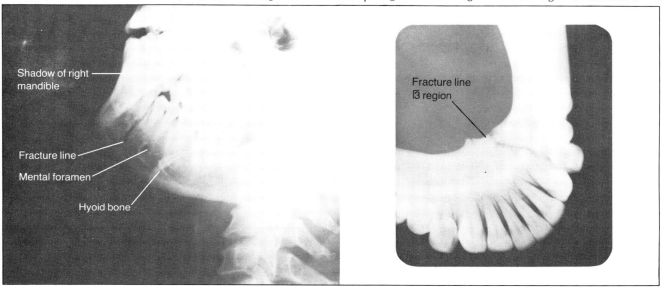

Shadow of right mandible

Fracture line

Mental foramen

Hyoid bone

Fracture line ⌐3 region

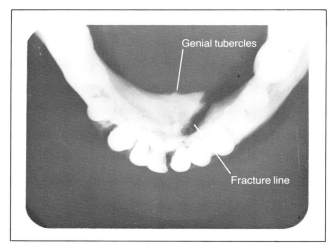

Figure 187. *A true lower occlusal view shows fracture of the midline extending to the lower border just left of the genial tubercles. Muscles have pulled the larger fragment, which includes the tubercles, inwards.*

Fractures of the middle third of the face can be divided into:

1. Alveolar.
2. Le Fort I.
3. Le Fort II.
4. Le Fort III.
5. Zygomatic arch.
6. Zygomatic complex.
7. Orbital 'blow-out'.
8. Nasal complex.

Alveolar Fractures

Fractures of the alveolar bone in the maxilla are more frequent than those of the mandibular alveolus. They generally arise in the anterior region as the direct result of a blow, and are often accompanied by subluxation,

Figure 188. *Fracture across the symphysis showing wide radiolucent fracture line and some displacement of fragments. Other views are required to show the displacement in a different plane.*

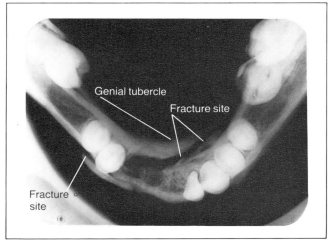

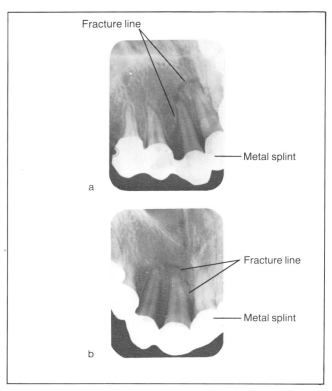

Figure 189. *The periapical radiographs 5-1| region show alveolar fracture line extending from the bone ridge crest between 1|1, above the apices 21| to the crest of the ridge anterior to 4| in this girl aged 20 years. 3| is missing. The cap splint immobilizes the anterior teeth until union takes place.*

dislocation, avulsion or fracture of the teeth in the area concerned. Figure 189 shows fracture of the alveolar process from the midline to the alveolar crest anterior to the first premolar. The canine would appear to be missing.

The maxillary tuberosity sometimes breaks away during attempted removal of the upper third molar, much to the chagrin of the operator. A radiograph taken before complete removal may help to make the

Figure 190. *Intraoral film of a man aged 24 years shows fracture of the left tuberosity to include |7. The shadow of the left coronoid process can be seen across the posterior part of the tuberosity.*

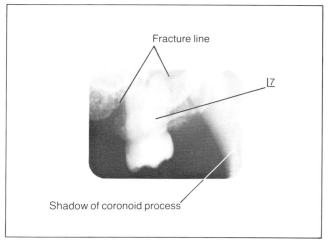

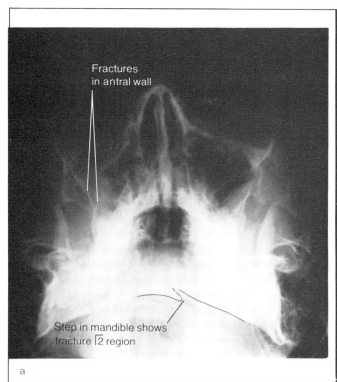

Fractures in antral wall

Step in mandible shows fracture ⌐2 region

a

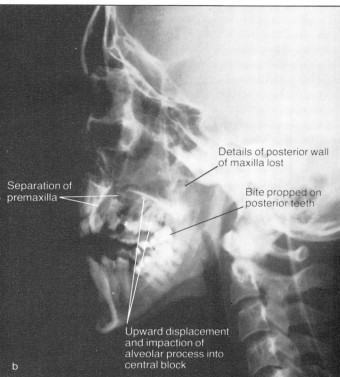

Separation of premaxilla

Details of posterior wall of maxilla lost

Bite propped on posterior teeth

Upward displacement and impaction of alveolar process into central block

b

decision as to whether to remove the bone and suture to avoid oroantral fistula, or whether to retain the tooth to act as a splint until the fracture has united, and then remove the tooth surgically. Figure 190 shows fracture of the left maxillary tuberosity as the result of a direct blow to this area.

Le Fort I Fractures

The Le Fort I, low-level fracture (Plate 1a and b) involves the lateral walls of the nose medially and the lateral walls of the antra laterally. Plate 1a shows the fracture line passing from the lateral wall of the nasal fossa above the canine eminence and below the zygomatic process along the lateral wall of the antrum. Plate 1b shows the fracture line continuing backwards across the tuberosity and involving the pterygoid plates. The fracture line across the tuberosity is continuous with that passing along the lateral wall of the nose.

The fracture can be unilateral, bilateral, or on both sides and down the midline suture. There may be considerable mobility of the detached toothbearing portion. Without displacement it is very difficult to see the lines of this fracture, as is evident in Figure 191a. Figure 191b, a true lateral skull radiograph shows a complete low transverse fracture of the alveolar process of the maxilla. There is upward displacement and impaction into the central block, and associated separation of the premaxilla. The marked propping of the bite posteriorly is obvious, and the posterior wall of the maxilla cannot be distinguished at all easily.

Figure 192 shows some of the angulations used in the occipitomental positionings to show fractures of the middle third of the face.

Figure 191 (a). *Occipitomental view of a man aged 27 years showing fractures of the lateral walls of the antra. The rest of the Le Fort I lines are not evident on this radiograph. The patient also has fracture of ⌐2 region (which can be seen as a step in the lower border of the mandible) and fracture of both condyles.* **(b)** *True lateral skull radiograph showing low-level Le Fort I fracture. There has been upward displacement and impaction of the alveolar process of the maxilla, and an associated separation of the premaxilla.*

Figure 192. *Radiographic positioning for occipitomental views of the jaws. 1. Standard occipitomental. Outer canthus of eye to external auditory meatus is at 45° to the horizontal. The central ray is projected horizontally. 2. 15° occipitomental. The central ray is projected downwards at 15°. Head is in same position as for standard occipitomental. 3. 30° occipitomental. The central ray is projected downwards at 30°. Head is in same position as for standard occipitomental.*

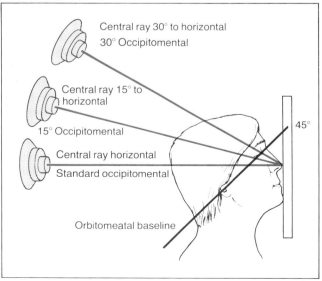

Central ray 30° to horizontal
30° Occipitomental

Central ray 15° to horizontal
15° Occipitomental

Central ray horizontal
Standard occipitomental

45°

Orbitomeatal baseline

Le Fort II Fractures

The Le Fort II subzygomatic fracture is pyramidal in shape (Plate 2a and b). The fracture line runs across the nasal bones laterally to cross the frontal process of the maxilla (which might present as a small 'step' in the medial wall of the orbit), through the lacrimal bones to cross the inferior border of the orbit, and drops down to the lateral wall of the antrum close to the zygomatic process (Plate 2a). This part of the fracture line's course is closely related to the zygomaticomaxillary suture. The fracture line then travels along the lateral wall of the antrum (Plate 2b) to cross the pterygomaxillary fissure and the pterygoid plates. The zygomatic complex may not be involved in this type of fracture.

Figure 193a, b and c shows a complete pyramidal fracture of the centre block of the face. There is little, if any, displacement of this block. In addition the patient has suffered a Le Fort I fracture, and the alveolar segment of the maxilla has been displaced backwards about $\frac{1}{4}$ in, and impacted slightly into the main block. Due to the lack of posterior teeth the usual propped bite is not obvious.

Le Fort III Fractures

The Le Fort III suprazygomatic, or high level, fracture separates the middle third of the face from the cranium (Plate 3a and b). The fracture line starts around the 'nasion' (Plate 3a), crosses the nasal, lacrimal bones and orbital part of the ethmoid to the vicinity of the orbital foramen (Plate 3b). Fortunately the ring of dense bone surrounding this foramen is seldom involved in the fracture line. From the medial aspect of the inferior orbital fissure the fracture line descends across the posterior portion of the maxilla high up and across the pterygomaxillary fissure to involve the pterygoid plates.

Figure 193 (a). *True lateral skull radiograph showing pyramidal fracture line extending from the region of the nasal bones, passing downwards and backwards. The nasal bones are comminuted and depressed. There is a large horizontal displacement of the posterior maxillary wall of the alveolar segment which is quite obvious.* **(b)** *10° occipitomental view showing fracture lines: horizontally across the nasal bones; in the left orbital floor (hardly evident); and low down in the lateral walls of both antra. The mandibular fracture in $\lceil 3$ region is evident by the vertical displacement of the over-riding fragments.* **(c)** *30° occipitomental view showing fracture of the nasal complex; the floor of the left orbit; and the lateral walls of both antra. The zygomatic arches appear intact. The displacement of $\lceil 3$ with respect to $\lceil 2$ is evident.*

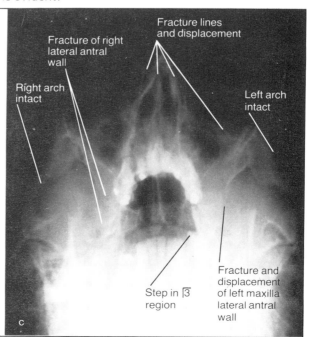

Fracture line of Le Forte II with little displacement

Marked displacement of posterior wall of maxilla

Comminution and depression of nasal profile

Frontal sinus

Fracture and displacement

Opaque antrum

Fracture of lateral wall right antrum

Intact arch

Fracture and slight displacement

Opaque part of antrum

Intact arch

Fracture lateral wall of left antrum

Displacement upwards of $\lceil 3$, due to fracture of mandible

Fracture lines and displacement

Fracture of right lateral antral wall

Right arch intact

Left arch intact

Step in $\lceil 3$ region

Fracture and displacement of left maxilla lateral antral wall

In addition there is a fracture line crossing the lateral wall of the orbit separating the frontal and the zygomatic bone, the zygomatic arch also being involved.

Figure 194a, b and c are true lateral, posteroanterior and occipitomental views showing a Le Fort III fracture. There is a complete high transverse fracture, and associated fractures of the temporal processes of the zygomatic arches, though these have maintained their normal curve.

Fractures of the Zygomatic Arch

Fractures of the zygomatic arch usually arise as the result of a direct blow to this part of the face, and Figure 195 illustrates a depressed fracture of the zygomatic arch on the patient's left side. The rest of the zygomatic complex appears normal. Figure 196 shows a comminuted fracture of the left zygomatic arch. There is also a fracture of the zygomatic complex, and a mucosal retention cyst of the right antrum.

Fractures of the Zygomatic Complex

The occipitomental projection shown in Figure 197 illustrates the four points at which fracture usually occurs in the zygomatic complex:

1. The zygomatic arch at the zygomaticotemporal suture region.
2. The zygomaticofrontal suture.
3. The floor of the orbit.
4. The lateral wall of the antrum.

Figure 194 (a). *True lateral skull view showing comminuted fracture of the nasal bones, and high transverse fracture through the zygomatico-frontal sutures and frontal bone. Also evident is disorganisation of the posterior walls of the maxilla. There is a complete transverse fracture of the alveolar process of the maxilla, which has been impacted into the central block with some displacement upwards and backwards.* **(b)** *Posteroanterior view showing the high transverse fracture well.* **(c)** *10° occipitomental view showing splints and fixation in place. This view also shows the fracture lines of the left orbital floor, left antral wall, right zygomatic arch, zygomaticofrontal suture line and nasal bones.*

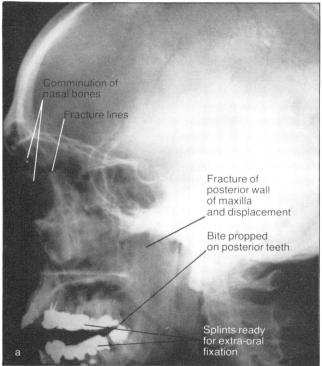

Comminution of nasal bones

Fracture lines

Fracture of posterior wall of maxilla and displacement

Bite propped on posterior teeth

Splints ready for extra-oral fixation

a

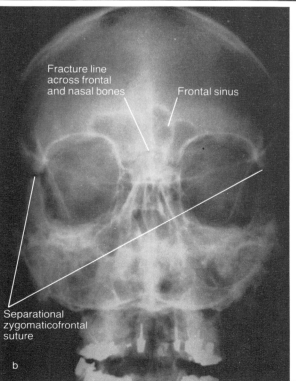

Fracture line across frontal and nasal bones

Frontal sinus

Separational zygomaticofrontal suture

b

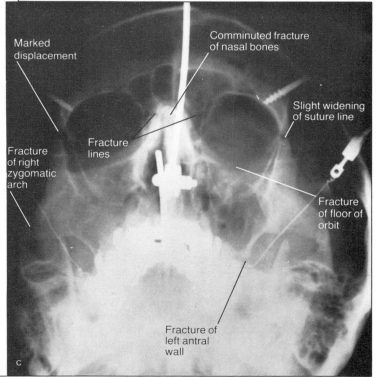

Marked displacement

Comminuted fracture of nasal bones

Slight widening of suture line

Fracture lines

Fracture of right zygomatic arch

Fracture of floor of orbit

Fracture of left antral wall

c

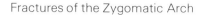

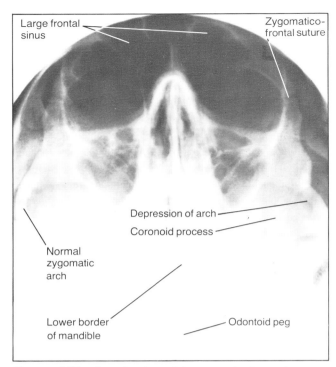

Figure 195. *Standard occipitomental view of a man aged 34 years showing depressed fracture of the left zygomatic arch. There is also slight opening of the zygomaticofrontal suture.*

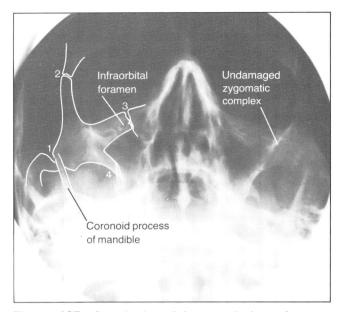

Figure 197. *Standard occipitomental view of a man aged 53 years showing depressed fracture of the right zygomatic complex and misalignment of the zygomatic arch. Numbered arrows point to the four typical fracture sites: 1. Zygomaticotemporal suture region; 2. Zygomaticofrontal suture region; 3. Floor of the orbit; 4. Lateral wall of the antrum. There is no suggestion of fracture of the left side.*

The fracture seen in Figure 197 is a depressed fracture of the zygoma. There is little opacity of the right antrum. Opacity of the related antrum is generally a marked feature of such fractures.

'Blow-out' Fractures of the Orbit

Fractures of the orbital rim usually occur in Le Fort II and III, and zygomatic complex fractures as a result of trauma to the various bones of the face. It is said that a

Figure 196. *Standard occipitomental view of a man aged 54 years showing comminuted fracture of the left zygomatic arch with the fragments seemingly in good alignment. The left antrum is completely opaque and this to some extent obscures the fracture of the left zygomatic complex, though depression of the outer third of the lower orbital rim can be seen. There is a mucosal retention cyst evident on the floor of the right antrum.*

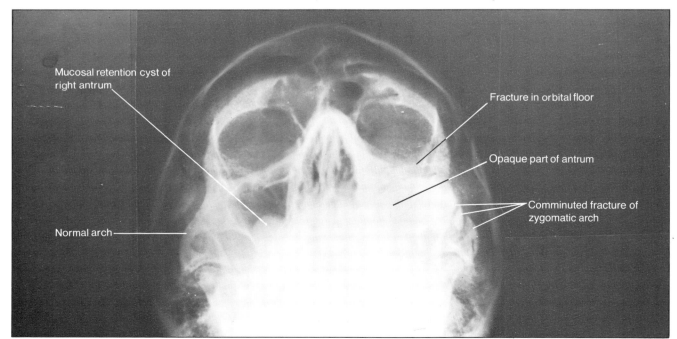

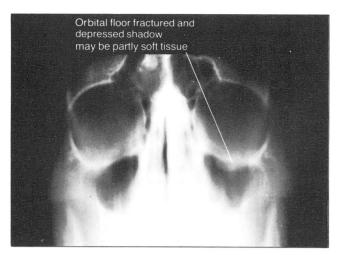

Figure 198. *Tomographic projection, occipitomental positioning, of a boy aged 16 years who had experienced a direct blow to the left eye. A displaced plate of the floor of the orbit can be seen in this radiograph (though this might conceivably just be a soft tissue hernia of the orbital contents).*

Figure 199. *True lateral projection with reduced exposure showing the nasal complex. There is evidence of fracture of the nasal bones in this radiograph.*

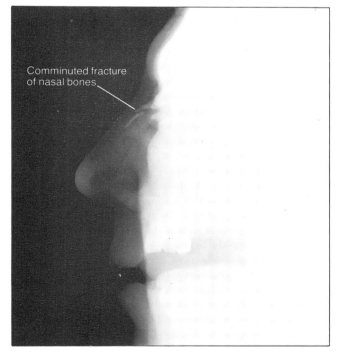

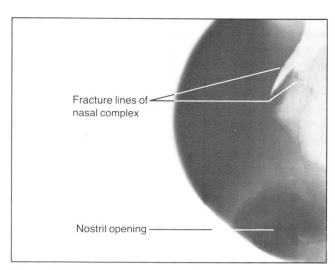

Figure 200. *Wrapped occlusal film held laterally beside the face showing fracture of the nasal bones, part of the bridge of the nose being bent downwards.*

direct blow to the eye itself, rather than to the surrounding orbit, may cause the orbital 'blow-out' fracture (Figure 198). Pressure to the eyeball is transmitted to the thin bone of the inferior wall of the orbit, and this is forced downwards. Figure 198 is a tomogram showing the inferior plate of bone, or orbital contents, pushed downwards from the orbit in a boy of 16 years following a direct blow to the left eye. The orbital rim appears to be intact, though clinically the eye itself was depressed somewhat and had little range of movement.

It has also been suggested that flexibility of the zygomatic complex may transmit the pressures of trauma through to the infraorbital wall, resulting in fracture of this plate rather than the orbital rims, the latter protecting the eyeball itself from damage. According to Campbell (1977), 20 per cent of 'blow-out' fractures occur through the orbital plate of the ethmoids.

Fractures of the Nasal Bones

This fairly frequent type of fracture is best shown on a true lateral projection. With the radiation considerably reduced, a true lateral view will outline the nasal bones clearly (Figure 199). An alternative is to use an occlusal film held against the side of the patient's face. Using a wrapped film the detail will be excellent. Figure 200 shows fracture of the nasal bones.

Reference

Worth, H. M., *Principles and Practice of Oral Radiologic Interpretation,* Year Book Medical Publishers Inc., Chicago, Ill., 1963.
Campbell, W., *Radiological Evaluation of Facial Fractures,* Weekly Radiology Science Update. No. 40, Biomedia Inc., Radiology Science Update Division, Pennsylvania, 1977.

5. Periapical Changes

'Look for the lamina' is probably the best advice a dental radiologist can give to students when dealing with the subject of periapical changes. This thimble of dense bone surrounding the tooth root is the most significant structure of the periapical tissues and accurate assessment of changes in its condition will generally enable a diagnosis to be made.

Radiographic evidence alone is insufficient, however, and vitality tests and clinical observation of the area under consideration, together with an assessment of the patient's general state of health, are of major importance in making a diagnosis.

General Considerations

Teeth can be dead and infected without there being any evidence of periapical change on the radiograph, or they can be very much alive and yet show an area of radiolucency. There may be radiolucent or opaque bone changes evident at the apices, or a combination of both. Resorption may or may not occur, and this may be internal or external.

There is a wide variation in the appearance of the outline of periapical lesions, and diagnosis is by no means obvious in all cases.

Histological investigation has shown that there are a number of normal structures, such as foramina, sparse trabeculation, calculi and dense bone islands, that can confuse the interpreter and lead to a false diagnosis from the radiographs. The study of apical change is a complex matter requiring careful consideration.

Periapical Radiography

Good radiographs, preferably intraoral views using the paralleling technique, are essential for periapical assessment. Foreshortening of the image by incorrect technique may result in early areas of bone change being missed. Even with excellent radiographs, small areas of bone change buccal or palatal to the roots of the teeth may not be seen, due to superimposition of the opacity of the root. The detail on extraoral views is not good enough in many instances to make a reliable diagnosis of early periapical change, and it is advisable in such cases to take further periapical radiographs intraorally.

Periapical Rarefaction

Generally, rarefaction of bone at the apex of a tooth arises as a result of death of the pulp and extension of the infection into the periapical tissues. It is quite possible, however, for the pulp to die, remain symptomless, and produce no periapical change, the lamina remaining intact. Figure 201 illustrates ⌊1 in a boy aged 14 years. This tooth was discoloured but symptomless, and there was a history of trauma one year previously. On investigation the tooth was found to be non-vital, though the radiographs show no sign of periapical change.

Varying Appearance of Radiolucencies

Early apical change can be seen as thinning of the lamina and widening of the periodontal membrane. Acute abscess may present with no radiographic evidence of periapical change, yet swelling and pain are present clinically. Sometimes there is a slight widening of the periodontal membrane shadow, due to the tissue fluid present forcing the tooth a little out of the socket.

Figure 202 shows early periapical change at the apex 7⌉ with loss of continuity of the lamina dura at the apex. There was a history of pain from this tooth.

Areas of rarefaction may increase in size until they appear to involve adjacent teeth (Figure 203). It is advisable to test all teeth in the neighbourhood for vitality as there have been instances of apparently unsuccessful root treatments where the adjacent tooth has turned out to be dead, thereby preventing the original area from healing. In Figure 203, ⌊123 have lost lamina and ⌊2 has had some external resorption distally on the root. The Y-line of Ennis landmark is well shown.

Figure 204 shows a fairly extensive diffuse area of bone change at the apex 2⌋. There is no obvious outline to the lesion, which has an 'invasive' look. There was no history of trauma in this instance. No filling is evident, neither is there any sign of caries. The large invaginated cingulum pit has led to food packing and death of the pulp.

Often the outlines of radiolucent areas are more definite (Figure 205), and there is the temptation to label such conditions as granuloma. It is not possible to do

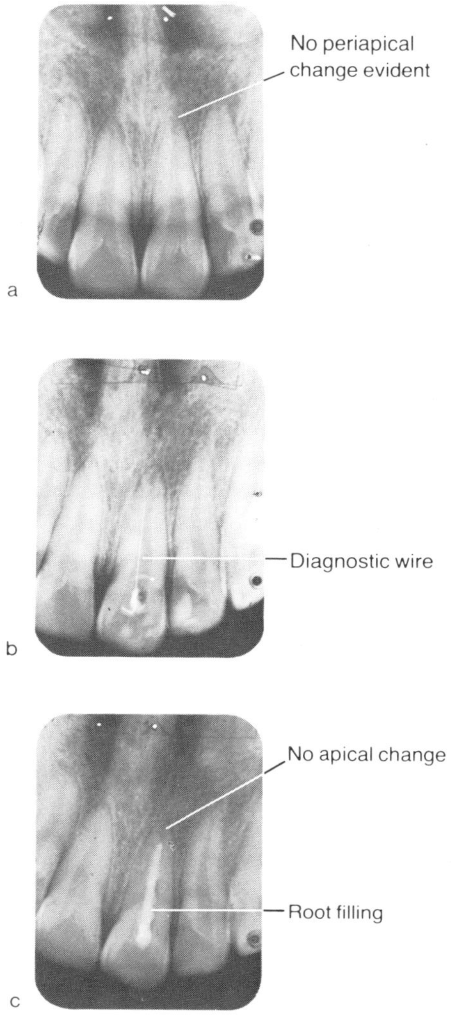
No periapical change evident
a
Diagnostic wire
b
No apical change
Root filling
c

Figure 201. *|1 was found to have a dead pulp, although no apical changes were evident on the radiograph, following a change in colour two years after trauma. The lamina dura has remained intact throughout.*

Figure 202. *Periapical radiograph showing early bone changes in 7|. The lamina has been eroded at the apices.*

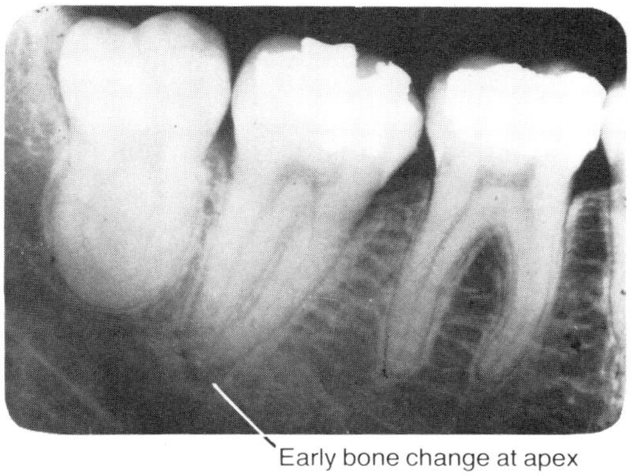
Early bone change at apex

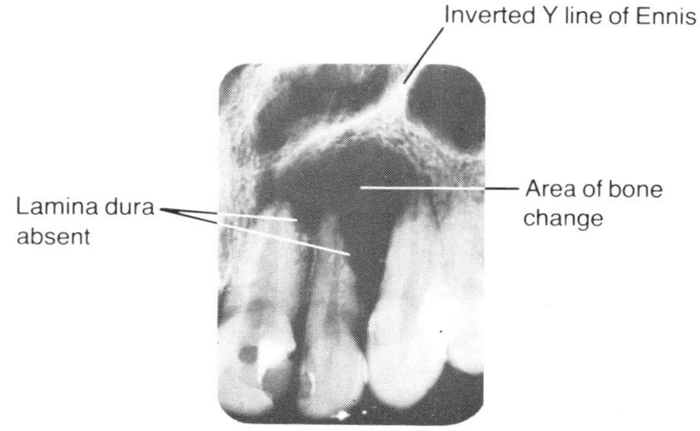
Inverted Y line of Ennis
Lamina dura absent
Area of bone change

Figure 203. *Periapical radiograph showing large radiolucent area of bone change centred on the apex of |2. Both |13 have lost some lamina, and |2 has had slight resorption of the apex. The inverted Y-line of Ennis shows well on the radiograph.*

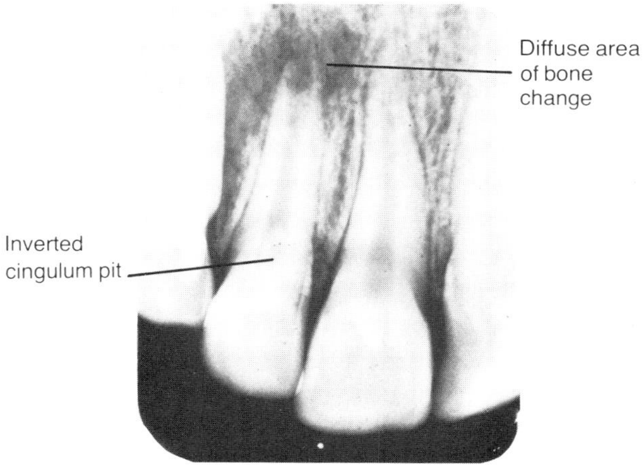
Diffuse area of bone change
Inverted cingulum pit

Figure 204. *Periapical radiograph of 2| region showing irregularly-outlined area of radiolucency over the root apex. The lamina is missing and a deep cingulum pit is evident.*

Figure 205. *Discrete circumscribed area of bone change at the apex of 2|, suggesting a granuloma to be present. There is an unlined filling evident in the tooth.*

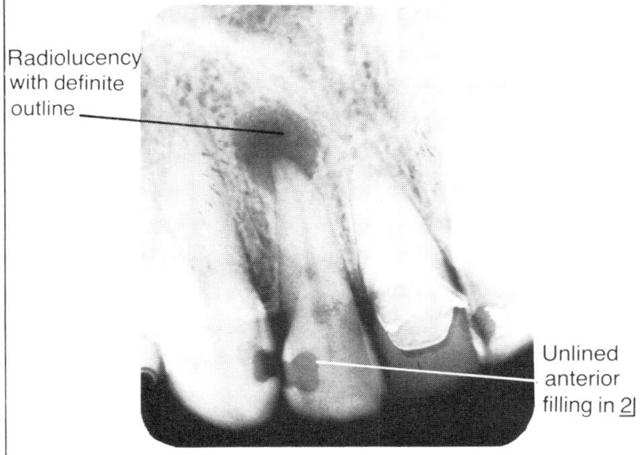
Radiolucency with definite outline
Unlined anterior filling in 2|

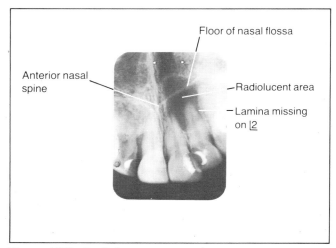

Figure 206. *Radiolucent area on* ⌊2 *suggestive of cyst. There is a thin cortical outline. A lamina is visible at the apex of* ⌊1.

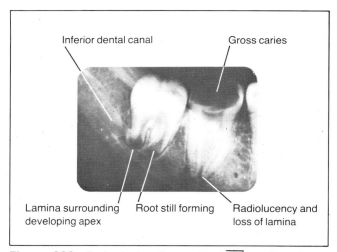

Figure 208. *Periapical radiograph of* 87̄⌉ *region showing developing roots of* 8⌉ *and early radiolucency at the apex* 7̄⌉. *The lamina surrounds the radiolucent radicular papillae of* 8⌉ *and is missing at the apex of* 7̄⌉.

this from the radiographic appearance, as early cyst or chronic abscess are just as likely. It is probable that this tooth died as a result of irritation of the pulp from the unlined filling distally.

The large radiolucent area centred on ⌊2 (Figure 206) appears to have a cortical margin and looks cystic in nature. It could, however, just as easily be a granuloma.

Deciduous Teeth

Single rooted teeth of the deciduous dentition produce areas of bone change at the apices which are sometimes hard to see because of the closeness of the crypts and crowns of the unerupted permanent teeth (Figure 209).

In the primary molar region bone changes often take place at the bifurcation of the roots (Figure 207). The

large size of the pulp and the presence of secondary canals running from the base of the pulp chamber to the bifurcation are the reasons for areas developing at this site. These areas may be missed as they can easily be mistaken for the crypt of the adjacent developing permanent tooth. Again, the lamina should be assessed carefully. In Figure 207 it is missing on the inside of the roots and at the bifurcation. In addition, there is a large carious cavity suggesting exposure of the pulp in D̄⌉.

Developing Teeth

A differential diagnosis must be made between developing teeth whose roots are incomplete, and permanent teeth with early bone change at the apices. Figure 208 shows both conditions. 8̄⌉ roots are incomplete; the

Figure 207. *Radiograph of* D̄⌉ *region showing radiolucent area at the bifurcation of the roots. The lamina dura is missing on the inside of the roots from the bifurcation to the apices.*

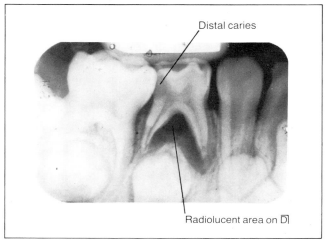

Figure 209. *Radiograph of a boy aged 7 years showing exfoliating* 4⌋. *The bone of the crypt has been destroyed.* C⌋ *is carious and appears to have an area of bone change at the apex, though this is difficult to see because of the proximity of the permanent lateral incisor and its crypt.*

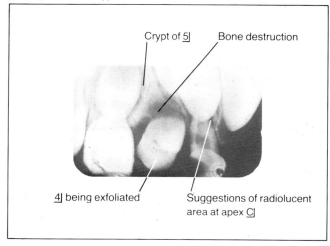

lamina dura surrounds the radicular papillae and is intact. These incomplete root ends cannot be confused with resorbing root ends as the deficiency is not only in the length of the roots, but also on the inside of the forming apices. In cases of resorption, the process would be mainly on the outside of the end of the root. The lower right second molar in Figure 208 has areas of radiolucency at the apices, and the lamina dura is missing at these points.

The crypt of a developing permanent tooth may become involved with an abscess on a primary tooth. There are three possible outcomes:

1. The infection will clear and the permanent tooth develops normally.

2. The infection causes hypoplasia of the permanent tooth resulting in a 'Turner tooth'.

3. The developing permanent tooth will be exfoliated.

Figure 209 illustrates exfoliation of 4| crown in a boy aged seven years. There has been bone destruction around the crypt and loss of the surrounding lamina. The outline of the radiolucent area is indefinite (compare with 5| crypt). In addition, there is the suggestion of a loss of lamina at the apex C|, though this is difficult to see because the crypt and crown of the permanent tooth lie directly above.

Orthodontic Treatment

Movement of teeth with appliance therapy has an effect upon the periapical tissues, and the results can sometimes be seen on radiographs.

Figure 210 shows |1 with an irregularly-bordered area of radiolucency at the apex and loss of the lamina. This girl, aged 11 years, had a sinus with a gumboil pointing between |12, and |1 was loose. Orthodontic treatment was in progress to retract |1 (not for the first time) with a removable appliance. Because of the radiographic appearance, |1 was opened palatally, but surprisingly was found to be vital. As |2 might conceivably have been the cause of the trouble, this was investigated in the same manner—and also proved to be vital. At this stage, instructions were given for the orthodontic appliance to be left out of the mouth temporarily, and cement dressings were put in the palatal pits. Figure 210b shows the condition four months later. There has been considerable bone regeneration in |12 region; the sinus had gone and both teeth responded to vitality tests. Ten months later (Figure 210c) there was a normal periapical bone pattern evident with a reformed lamina across the apex of |1. There is the suggestion of minimal resorption at the apex of this tooth. Both |12 were vital and firm, and the palatal pits were filled with amalgam.

Periodontal Bone Loss to Apex

Periodontal disease can result in loss of most of the intraradicular bone (Figure 211a). It can also progress

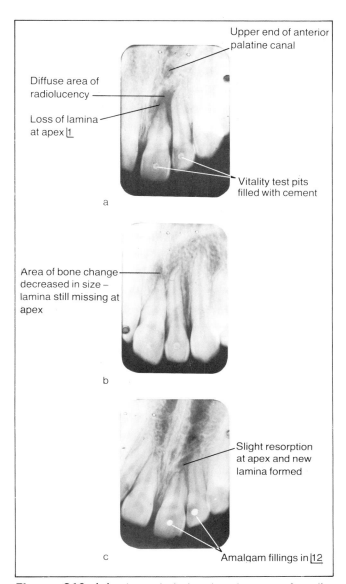

Figure 210 (a). *Irregularly-bordered area of radiolucency at the apex of |1 and loss of apical lamina in a girl aged 11 years who was wearing an orthodontic appliance. Both |12 were found to be vital, although there was a sinus pointing between them. Instructions were given for the plate to be left out.* (b) *Four months later the area had decreased considerably in size, and the sinus had gone.* (c) *A further 10 months later there is a normal periapical bone pattern and a reformed lamina dura across the apex of |1. There is some resorption. The tooth is vital and symptomless.*

to involve the apical region of the tooth (Figure 211b), though the latter may remain vital. In Figure 211b the lamina dura around the socket has been lost, and calculus, or small bony sequestra, are evident in the radiolucency mesial to the tooth on the original radiograph. The final picture may present as in Figure 211c, where there is no socket bone left and the tooth is held in by soft tissue only. The author has had the unusual experience of inadvertently removing a premolar with a probe whilst making a routine examination for a patient with gross periodontal disease. It was difficult to say who was the more surprised by the painless extraction.

Apart from an haematogenous infection carried from a focus elsewhere in the body, osteomyelitis (a spreading infection of bone) may arise in the jaws from infection following operative procedures and the extension of periapical infections. Lowered resistance of the host to infection is a predisposing factor. The mandible is more frequently involved than the maxilla, due to the relatively poor blood supply of the former.

Figure 212 shows the radiographic appearance of a patient aged 37 years who attended with a sinus pointing in the buccal aspect of the alveolar bone in ⌈3 region. ⌈4 root had been recently removed. There is a likely area of bone change at the apex of ⌈2 and the distal root of ⌈6 is suspicious. In due course ⌈23 were removed, following which the patient developed osteomyelitis (Figure 213), possibly as a result of the infection already present in ⌈4 region spreading forwards, but just as likely arising from the infection originally present at the apex of ⌈2. Large areas of radiolucency are evident and some sequestration. Seventeen days later healing was in progress, and the radiographs (Figure 214) show a periosteal reaction at the lower border of the mandible with formation of new bone in 1⌉123 region. The films also

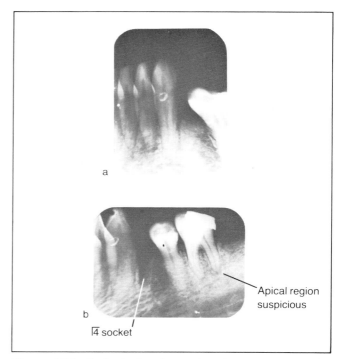

Figure 212. *Periapical radiographs of a woman aged 37 years showing periapical bone change on ⌈2 and ⌈6. The patient had a sinus pointing buccally on the alveolus in ⌈3 region. ⌈4 socket is evident on the posterior radiograph.*

a

b
⌈4 socket

Apical region suspicious

indicate that though sequestra are still present a number have been discharged. The apices of ⌈6 are still doubtful, but in the circumstances it was probably as well that this tooth had not been extracted!

Figure 211 (a). *A loss of supporting bone includes the septum between the roots of 7⌉, and reaches down to the apex.* **(b)** *Bone loss has reached the apex of this tooth with complete loss of lamina. Small spicules of bone or calculus can be seen mesial to 7⌉.* **(c)** *There is no supporting bone left for ⌊6. It is maintained in position by soft tissue.*

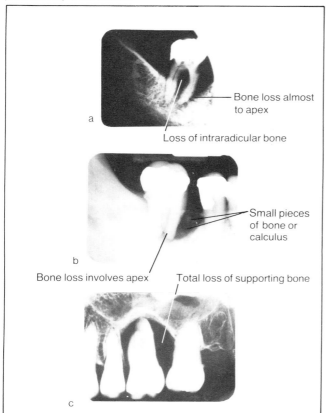

a
Bone loss almost to apex

Loss of intraradicular bone

b
Small pieces of bone or calculus

Bone loss involves apex

Total loss of supporting bone

c

Figure 213. *The same patient as Figure 212 after removal of ⌈23. A wide area of bone has been destroyed and sequestra can be seen. This is the spreading infection of osteomyelitis.*

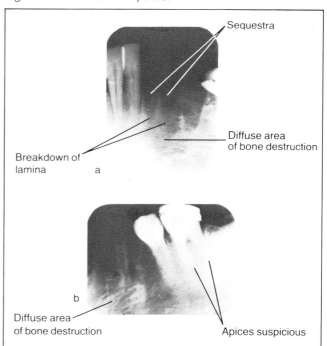

Sequestra

Breakdown of lamina

a

Diffuse area of bone destruction

b

Diffuse area of bone destruction

Apices suspicious

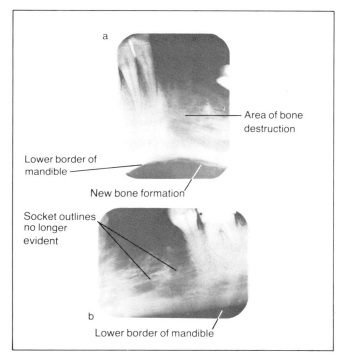

Figure 214. *The same patient as Figure 213 17 days later. Some sequestra are still evident and some have been discharged. There is new bone formation at the lower border of the mandible in 1⌐123 region. The apex of ⌐6 is still suspicious.*

Resorption

Internal or external resorption may occur following trauma or irritation from unlined anterior filling materials, followed by death of the tooth and development of a periapical area. Figure 215, a periapical view of ⌐2 region of an 11-year-old boy, illustrates such a case. Figure 216 shows an old fracture of 2⌐ in a man aged 36 years, where there has been some resorption of the fractured root ends and internal resorption nearer to the pulp chamber. The bone at the end of the true apex appears to be sound.

Figure 215. *Periapical radiograph of ⌐2 region of a boy aged 11 years. ⌐3 apex is incomplete. There is internal resorption and an area of radiolucency at the apex. The lamina is missing too.*

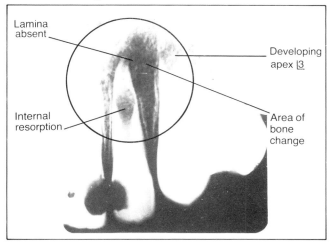

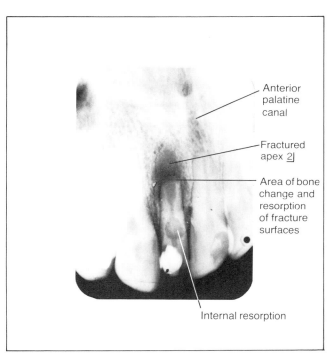

Figure 216. *Radiograph of a man aged 36 years showing old fracture of the root of 2⌐. There has been some resorption of the fractured root ends, though the true apex appears sound. The radiolucency between the fracture ends could signify infection. There has been internal resorption in the coronal root fragment.*

'Residual' Radiolucencies

On occasions the removal of an offending tooth may not result in clearance of infection, nor in complete removal of a granuloma or cyst. Figure 217a is a

Figure 217 (a). *A periapical radiograph 6-2⌐ region of a 44-year-old man showing radiolucent areas of residual infection.* **(b)** *The same patient showing a residual area of radiolucency reminiscent of cyst in ⌐2 region.*

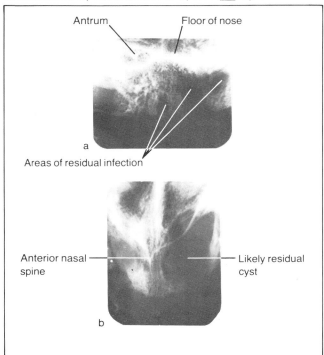

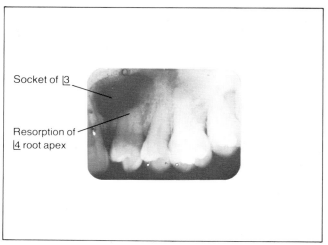

Figure 218. *Bone defect in a man aged 40 years resulting from removal of unerupted $\lfloor$3. There is pressure resorption of $\lfloor$4 apex. The area could be mistaken for a cyst or cleft.*

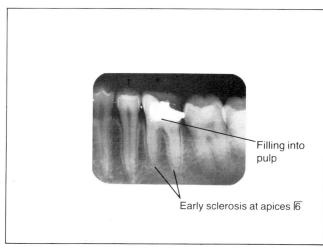

Figure 220. *Periapical radiograph of man aged 28 years showing mild sclerosis at apices $\lceil$6. The filling material was in contact with the pulp when investigated.*

radiograph of 6-2$\rfloor$ region of a man aged 44 years complaining of discomfort in the maxilla. Well-defined radiolucent areas suggestive of residual infection can be seen, though there is no evidence of sequestra present. Figure 217b is a midline view of the maxilla of the same patient, showing what appears to be a residual cyst in $\lfloor$2 region with a well-delineated outline.

These residual areas of bone change should not be confused with the radiolucency that results following the removal of an unerupted odontome or tooth. Figure 218 shows a bone defect, resulting from recent removal of a buried canine, which is somewhat suggestive of cyst. Some pressure resorption is evident at the apex of $\lfloor$4.

It should be borne in mind that, in the repair process, bone may not always fill the radiolucent region under consideration. The repair may be accomplished with the formation of fibrous tissue—the radiograph still showing the area to be radiolucent (Figure 219). In the event of there being no clinical signs of trouble, serial radiographs should be taken at yearly intervals, and these should show no enlargement of the area. Unnecessary repeat apicectomies have been done, in the mistaken belief that the first operation had failed, because of residual radiolucency evident six months to a year later on follow-up radiographs. In such cases it is advisable to test the adjacent teeth for vitality in case one of these was the cause of the original area.

Figure 219. *Periapical radiograph $\lfloor$2 region showing unerupted tooth or odontome in 1$\rfloor$ region. Also evident is failure of bone regeneration at the apex of resected root of $\lfloor$2 resulting in fibrous repair.*

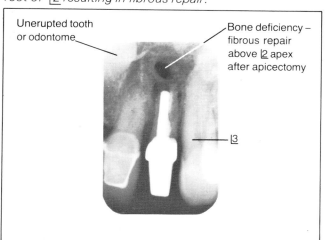

Figure 221. *Extensive mild sclerosis at the apices of root filled $\lceil$7. The lamina is absent at the apices. Amalgam waste from filling at the same visit can be seen resting in the buccal sulcus.*

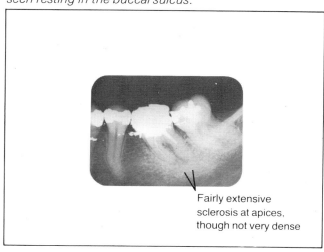

Sclerosing Osteitis

Sclerosing osteitis, which results in an increase in opacity at the apex of the tooth on the radiograph, may be caused by a low grade infection at the tooth apex. It may also result from the toxic products liberated from the infected pulp canal. The irritation causes osteoblasts to lay down fresh bone along the trabeculations, thereby increasing the density. Figure 220 illustrates early apical sclerosis at the roots of ⌐6. The lining under the amalgam filling was in direct contact with the pulp, and the resulting irritation has resulted in the sclerotic reaction at the apex. Teeth can exhibit mild apical sclerosis and still give a vital response.

Larger areas of sclerosis may be of moderate density (Figure 221), or very dense, and in the latter case it may be difficult to differentiate true sclerosing osteitis from very dense bone (see Figure 230) or dense bone islands (Figure 60)—variations of normal anatomy. The presence of a lamina dura and a positive vitality test should settle the matter.

Sclerosing osteitis may enclose an area of radiolucency (Figure 222a to d). Sometimes it is difficult to tell whether the bone surrounding the radiolucent area is sclerotic or just normal dense bone (Figure 223), particularly if this is near the mylohyoid line.

A very slowly progressive lesion, such as a chronic alveolar abscess, may result in resorption of the associated apex with an area of sclerotic bone surrounding the rarefaction at the resorbing apices (Figure 224a and b).

Sinus Tract

Drainage may occur by way of a sinus, but it should not be assumed that the sinus always points opposite the tooth responsible. Figure 225 shows a GP point following the route of sinus which opened at the mesial aspect of 3⌐. The periodontist treating the patient as-

Figure 222 (a). *Apical sclerosis surrounding widened periodontal membrane space shadow at the mesial root of ⌐6.* **(b)** *Large radiolucent area at the apices 6⌐ surrounded by sclerosing osteitis. The lamina is absent at the apices, and there is bone loss reaching to the bifurcation. 8⌐ is unerupted.* **(c)** *Extensive radiolucency at the apices of 6⌐ with surrounding sclerosing osteitis. The condition appears to have reached the bifurcation and there is bone destruction there too. 8⌐ is horizontally impacted. There is not much sign of lamina dura generally — further radiographs and tests might be advantageous to eliminate the possibility of hyperparathyroidism.* **(d)** *Large radiolucent area at the mesial apex of 6⌐ surrounded by a zone of sclerotic bone. The distal root apex is also affected. Distal apex of 7⌐ is suspicious, especially as there is a large filling and caries evident. A vitality test is indicated.*

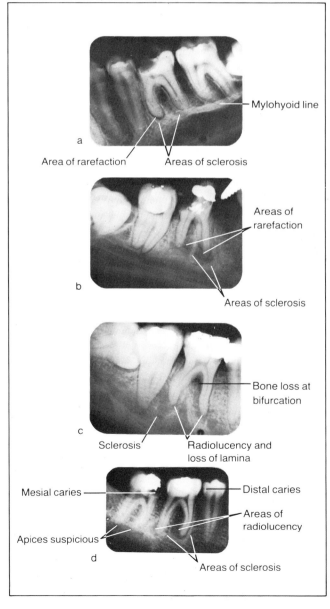

a — Mylohyoid line
Area of rarefaction — Areas of sclerosis

b — Areas of rarefaction — Areas of sclerosis

c — Bone loss at bifurcation — Sclerosis — Radiolucency and loss of lamina

d — Mesial caries — Distal caries — Apices suspicious — Areas of radiolucency — Areas of sclerosis

Figure 223. *Periapical radiograph shows radiolucent areas of bone change at the apices 6⌐. The bone above the mylohyoid line is dense generally, and it is difficult to say if there is sclerosis surrounding the radiolucencies. The periodontal membrane shadow at the apex of 8⌐ appears darker and wider than normal because of the overlying lucency of the mandibular canal. The tooth is vital.*

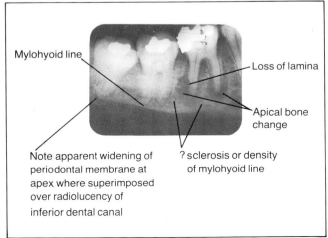

Mylohyoid line — Loss of lamina — Apical bone change — Note apparent widening of periodontal membrane at apex where superimposed over radiolucency of inferior dental canal — ? sclerosis or density of mylohyoid line

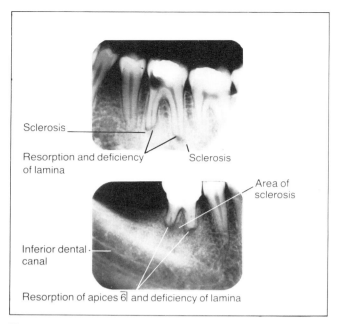

Sclerosis

Resorption and deficiency of lamina

Sclerosis

Area of sclerosis

Inferior dental canal

Resorption of apices 6⌐ and deficiency of lamina

Figure 224 (a) *Areas of radiolucency show at the resorbed apices of ⌐6. These are surrounded by areas of opacity. There is a large cavity mesially in this tooth.* **(b)** *There are small areas of rarefying osteitis at the resorbed apices of crowned 6⌐ in this woman aged 35 years. These areas are, in turn, surrounded by bone of increased density.*

sumed, quite correctly, that the lower canine was unlikely to be the cause, and the radiograph shows the GP point reaching the area of bone change at the apex of the root treated 4⌐. An amalgam 'tattoo' can be seen on the alveolar ridge in 6⌐ region.

The track of a sinus can seldom be seen on a radiograph unless there is a large tract leading to a marked perforation of the buccal or lingual plate of bone.

Figure 225. *This patient presented with a sinus in 32⌐ region on the buccal aspect of the alveolus. The GP point shows the tract and ends at the apex of the root filled 4⌐. There is no sign of lamina at the apex of this tooth and the date of the root filling would help in deciding the diagnosis and treatment planning. An amalgam 'tattoo' presents in 6⌐ region.*

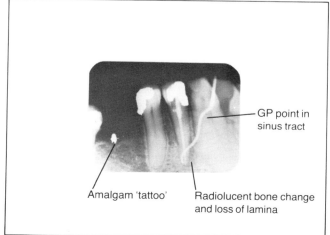

GP point in sinus tract

Amalgam 'tattoo'

Radiolucent bone change and loss of lamina

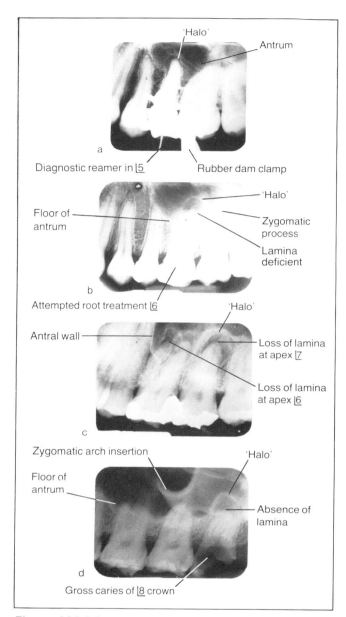

'Halo'

Antrum

a

Diagnostic reamer in ⌐5

Rubber dam clamp

Floor of antrum

'Halo'

Zygomatic process

Lamina deficient

b

Attempted root treatment ⌐6

'Halo'

Antral wall

Loss of lamina at apex ⌐7

Loss of lamina at apex ⌐6

c

Zygomatic arch insertion

'Halo'

Floor of antrum

Absence of lamina

d

Gross caries of ⌐8 crown

Figure 226 (a). *An opaque 'halo' can be seen over ⌐5. This is formed by periosteal lining of the antrum in advance of the radiolucent area of infection. The lamina is missing from ⌐5 apex.* **(b)** *'Halo' on ⌐6. The lamina is missing at the apex.* **(c)** *'Halo' on ⌐7. The lamina is missing at the apex.* **(d)** *'Halo' at the apex ⌐8. The lamina is missing at the apex.*

Antral 'Halo'

Acute infection at the apex of an upper premolar may be closely related to the antrum, and may result in a breakdown of the bone of the antral floor and sinusitis. A more chronic type of periapical infection will result in slow destruction of the bone of the antral floor, and stimulation of the periosteal lining of the antrum to lay down new bone ahead of the destruction. This results in a 'halo' of opaque bone above the rarefied area at the apex of the tooth (⌐5, ⌐6, ⌐7 and ⌐8 in Figure 226a to d). The lamina is absent from the apices of all teeth involved.

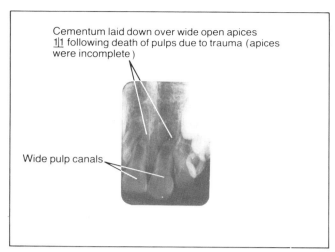

Figure 227. *Periapical radiograph of 1|12 region, showing cementum 'plugs' at the apices of 1|1 laid down by the body in an attempt to wall-off the dead pulps.*

Repair of Periapical Lesions

Removal of the tooth, or clearing the infection by root canal treatment will generally result in repair taking place. This may be by fibrous tissue (Figure 219), or by the formation of calcific material of varying density.

Sometimes cementum is laid down across the wide open apices of children's incisor teeth in the body's attempt to 'wall-off' dead pulps from the periapical tissues. Figure 227 illustrates this. Stimulation of the cementoblasts by irritation or infection may result in hypercementosis.

Root Canal Treatment

Root canal treatment, if undertaken with care, may result in complete repair of the periapical tissues, even though there may have been marked areas of bone change present initially (see Chapter 6).

In those cases where apical areas of bone change fail to respond to root canal treatment, or where root filling material has been forced through the apex, it may be necessary to resect the apex and clean out the infected bone.

Periapical Osteofibrosis

The radiographic appearance of these lesions at an early stage is highly suggestive of apical granuloma or infection. They most frequently appear at the apices of the lower anterior teeth (Figure 228a), but can occur at the apices of any of the permanent teeth. The writer has not seen this condition in the primary dentition. The aetiology of this bone-replacing fibrous tissue area is thought to be trauma, and a recent case of multiple periapical osteofibrosis, involving a number of teeth in both maxilla and mandible, presented in a 'cobbler' who held nails between his teeth throughout the day. The condition may remain static for many years, and sometimes resolves spontaneously, the apical bone re-

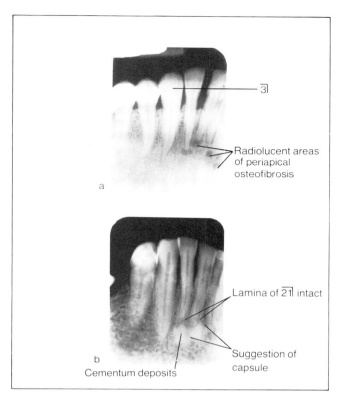

Figure 228 (a). *Radiolucent areas at the apices of the lower incisor teeth which are vital. This is the radiographic appearance of periapical osteofibrosis with no calcification.* **(b)** *Cementum can be laid down in the fibrous tissue matrix of periapical osteofibrosis to form an opacity such as is illustrated in this periapical radiograph.*

turning to normal with remodelling of the lamina dura. The lesion can increase in size, and in density as cementum is laid down in the fibrous matrix, giving at first a patchy opacity throughout the area. With completion of the process, an opacity with much the same density as dentine can be seen (Figure 228b). A capsule of fibrous tissue can often be seen surrounding the cementum with a clearcut outline. The most important investigation to make is a vitality test, as teeth with periapical osteofibrosis will give a positive response. No treatment is necessary, but serial radiographs at yearly intervals are advantageous.

Tumours

Tumours presenting in the alveolus can give rise to appearances not unlike cysts, granulomas and areas of periapical infection.

Figure 229 illustrates a benign giant cell lesion in |345 region in a woman aged 24 years. The premolar roots have been pushed aside and there is some deficiency of lamina around all three related teeth. There is no obvious root resorption, though this often does occur. The lobulated appearance helps to differentiate from a cyst.

Other tumours, such as ameloblastoma, can cause resorption and separation of the roots of adjacent teeth.

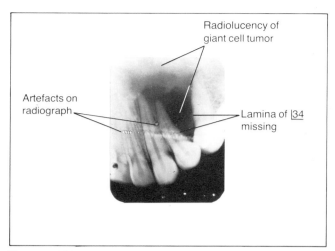

Figure 229. *Intraoral radiograph of ⌊4 region of a woman aged 24 years showing the radiolucent appearance of a giant-cell lesion. The roots of ⌊45 have been pushed apart and there is considerable loss of lamina around the teeth related to the lesion. There are also artefact marks on the radiograph.*

Confusion with Normal Anatomical Structures

Normal Bone

Areas of sparse trabeculation at the apices of teeth (Figure 230) can cause confusion with periapical lesions, and careful assessment of the lamina dura, together with the absence of fillings or caries, should eliminate the possibility of non-vital teeth. The figure also shows dense bone at the distal root ⌈6 which is a developmental abnormality. The periodontal membrane shadow can be seen and is normal.

Figure 231 is a periapical radiograph showing what might be cyst or ameloblastoma on 8⌉ which is partly

Figure 230. *Periapical radiograph of ⌈6 region showing sparse trabeculation between the apices of ⌈6. There is dense bone distally to this tooth which is a developmental abnormality. The periodontal membrane shadow can be seen surrounding the roots. The mesial apex of ⌈7 is highly suspicious, but the tooth was found to be vital.*

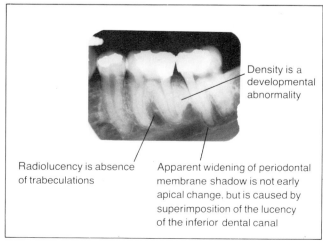

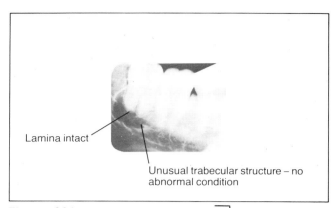

Figure 231. *Periapical radiograph 8⌉ shows what at first sight appears to be an apical cyst. It could be several other conditions, such as ameloblastoma or periodontal cyst. The lamina is intact. When 8⌉ was removed, no cyst cavity was evident. The pathology report stated: 'normal bone fragments; no epithelium evident'.*

impacted occlusally. On careful examination the lamina is seen to be intact—could it be a lateral periodontal cyst? The tooth was removed with surrounding tissue. No epithelium was found, neither did any cystic area materialize. The histological report was 'normal bone fragments; no epithelium'.

Foramina

The anterior palatine fossa and canal can cause diagnostic problems, as can the mental foramen. Figure 232a shows a radiolucent area at the apex of ⌊3. The tooth was non-vital. The anterior palatine canal can be seen running upwards, superimposed on the ⌊1. There is some apparent widening of the periodontal membrane at the apex of this tooth and gross bone loss. It is hard to decide from the radiograph alone whether or not there is an apical area.

Figure 232b shows a radiolucency at the apex of ⌊2 and loss of lamina. The large radiolucency adjacent to ⌊1 apex might be mistaken for an area on a lateral canal—but it is the anterior palatine fossa. The lamina dura is intact around ⌊1 and the tooth vital.

Figure 232c shows a radiolucency at the apex ⌊2 and early bone change at the apex ⌊1. Both teeth were dead on investigation.

Figure 232d is confusing. The sharply-outlined radiolucency seen above the arm of the spring cantelever bridge could be the anterior palatine fossa, residual infection, granuloma or cyst from ⌊1, or fibrous repair and deficiency of the buccal plate. A clinical examination and history taking are essential.

Figure 233a is an example of periapical infection at a premolar apex. This area should not be mistaken for the mental foramen, as the lamina dura is absent at the apex. Figure 233b shows a radiolucent area over the apex of ⌈5. This is the mental foramen as the lamina is intact.

Figure 233c shows a deficiency of lamina at the apex of carious ⌈4. There is the suggestion of loss of lamina

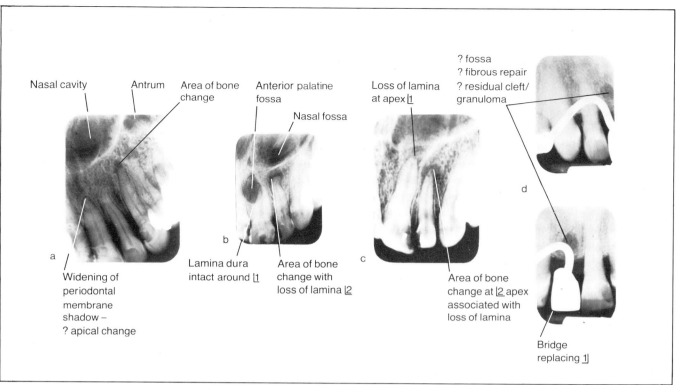

Nasal cavity   Antrum   Area of bone change

a

Widening of periodontal membrane shadow – ? apical change

Anterior palatine fossa

Nasal fossa

b

Lamina dura intact around |1

Area of bone change with loss of lamina |2

Loss of lamina at apex |1

c

Area of bone change at |2 apex associated with loss of lamina

? fossa
? fibrous repair
? residual cleft/ granuloma

d

Bridge replacing 1|

Figure 232, above (a). *Periapical radiograph of |3 region with radiolucent area of bone change at the apex of |3. The periodontal membrane at the apex |1 appears to be widened, and the anterior palatine fossa covers this area. Clinical investigation is necessary to make a diagnosis of non-vital |1.* **(b)** *There is a radiolucent area over |2 apex, which is the result of bone change. The radiolucent area at the apex of |1 in this 20-year-old man is the anterior palatine fossa as the lamina is intact.* **(c)** *The lamina is not intact over |12. Both these teeth are non-vital, though the apical condition of |1 might be missed by the large area on |2 producing 'tunnel vision' in the interpreter!* **(d)** *Intraoral radiographs showing a radiolucent area in 1| region. This could be an anterior palatine fossa, granuloma, cyst or fibrous repair! Follow-up radiographs in a year would be advantageous.*

Figure 233 (a). *Periapical radiograph showing area of radiolucency at the apex of root filled 4|. There is a surrounding area of sclerosing osteitis. The root filling is short and it is likely that infection is still present. The opacity in the alveolus distal to 4| is amalgam that probably fell into a tooth socket during the extraction.* **(b)** *Periapical radiograph of 5| region showing a radiolucent area at the apex of this tooth. There is an obvious lamina dura surrounding the root, so this radiolucency is the mental foramen.* **(c)** *Periapical radiograph of |4 region showing large area of bone change at the apex of this tooth which appears to involve |35 as well. There is lamina missing from all these teeth. The darker area within the large radiolucency represents the mental foramen, and in the original radiograph the mental canal can be seen running upwards and backwards towards this dark area. There is a large cavity in |4, but |3 has a sound crown and may well be vital. Vitality tests are required for |35.*

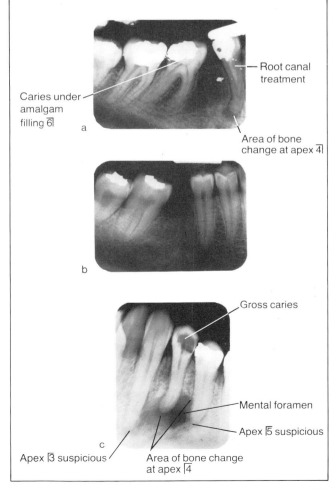

Caries under amalgam filling 6|

a

Root canal treatment

Area of bone change at apex 4|

b

Gross caries

Mental foramen

Apex |5 suspicious

c

Apex |3 suspicious

Area of bone change at apex |4

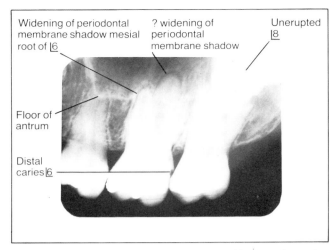

Widening of periodontal membrane shadow mesial root of ⌊6

? widening of periodontal membrane shadow

Unerupted ⌊8

Floor of antrum

Distal caries ⌊6

Figure 234. *Periapical radiographs of ⌊6 region of a woman aged 20 years. There is an unerupted ⌊8 evident. There is deep distal caries in ⌊6. In addition, there is widening of the periodontal membrane suggested at the apical parts of the anterobuccal and palatal roots superimposed on the maxillary antrum. The distobuccal root apex is not easy to determine on the radiograph. These apices could be within normal limits, but the periodontal membrane shadow is still wider than normal on the anterobuccal root below the level of the antral floor—and is therefore true widening. The radiographic report states: '⌊6 has deep distal caries and early periapical bone change'. A vitality test would confirm, or refute, the radiographic diagnosis.*

at ⌐5 root mesially. In the large radiolucent region between the two premolar roots is a small, darker, radiolucent well-defined area which is the mental foramen. The mental canal can be seen running upwards and backwards to reach this foramen.

Inferior Dental Canal and Maxillary Antrum

Superimposition of the apices of the lower molars on the inferior dental canal will often give the appearance of early bone change. The periodontal membrane shadow appears darker and wider than that part of the membrane superimposed on the opacity of the mylohyoid line (Figures 223 and 230). This sometimes makes it difficult to assess true early bone change at these molar apices.

The same appearance can be given at the apex of the palatal root of molars superimposed on the radiolucency of the antrum when using the bisected angle

technique. In Figure 234, the radiographic report reads: '⌊6 has deep distal caries and early periapical bone change'. This is correct, as the apparent widening of the periodontal membrane shadow on the mesial aspect of the anterobuccal root, where there is superimposition of the air sinus, continues below the level of the antral floor, suggesting true widening. The periodontal membrane of the palatal root appears to be widened at the apex, but this could be within normal limits. An unerupted ⌊8 can be seen in the corner of the radiograph.

Differential Diagnosis of Apical Changes

The main conditions and structures that may result in the projection of true or apparent radiolucent or radio-opaque periapical areas of bone change on radiographs are given in Table 1.

Table 1. The main conditions and structures that may result in the projection of true or apparent radiolucent or radio-opaque periapical areas of bone change on radiographs.

Apical radiolucencies
Acute abscess
Chronic abscess
Granuloma
Cyst
Tumour
Papilla of forming root
Periodontal abscess
Osteomyelitis
Haematoma
Area of sparse trabeculation
Thin bone in 2⌋2 regions
Fibrous repair
Periapical osteofibrosis
Shadow of *inferior dental* canal over apices
Shadow of foramina over apices
Shadow of antra over apices

Apical sclerosis
Sclerosing osteitis resulting from infection
Sclerosing osteitis resulting from toxins from pulp
Dense bone islands
Odontomes
Superimposed calculi
Cementoma and similar tumours
Paget's disease—second stage
Fibrous dysplasia
Overlying mylohyoid line
Artefacts on panoramic views, e.g. opaque earring shadows

6. Resorption, and Root Canal Treatment

Resorption

Resorption of teeth is either physiological, or arises as a result of some abnormal condition or force. Radiographs are helpful in determining the extent of resorption, but intraoral views are essential as screen film produces a rather blurred image—particularly when used with panoramic machines.

Physiological Resorption of Primary Teeth

Generally, physiological resorption is accepted as meaning the shortening of tooth roots of the primary dentition prior to their natural exfoliation. The process is usually fairly even across the width of the roots (Figures 235 and 236a). It may occur more extensively on one of the molar roots leaving the other root almost intact (Figure 236b and c). The process of resorption may continue well into the crown until very little coronal material is left (Figure 237), and yet the residue is still retained in position.

On occasions resorption is instigated by unerupted permanent teeth placed mesially or distally to the resorbing tooth, rather than by the teeth directly below (Figure 238). In this figure the mesial aspects of the anterior roots of $\overline{D|D}$ appear to be resorbing due to the close proximity of $\overline{3|3}$.

Figure 236 (a). *Right bitewing radiograph of a boy aged 9 years. There is even resorption of both roots of $\overline{D|}$. (**b**) Left bitewing radiograph of the same patient as (a) showing extensive resorption of the distal root of $\overline{|D}$ and little resorption of the mesial root. (**c**) Left bitewing radiograph of a girl aged 8½ years showing well-resorbed distal root of $\overline{|E}$ and less-resorbed mesial root. $\overline{|D}$ roots have even resorption.*

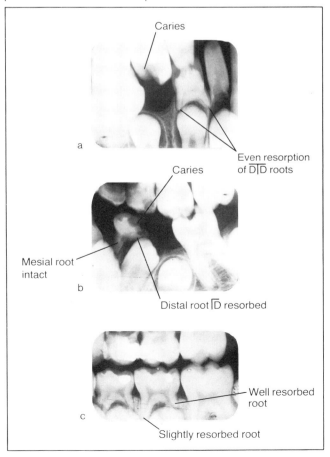

Figure 235. *Part of a standard occlusal radiograph showing physiological resorption of $\underline{A|A}$ in this boy aged 8 years. As expected there is no lamina across the resorbing root ends. Following earlier trauma the pulp of $\underline{A|}$ has calcified.*

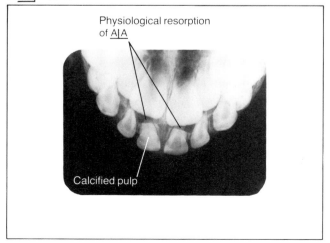

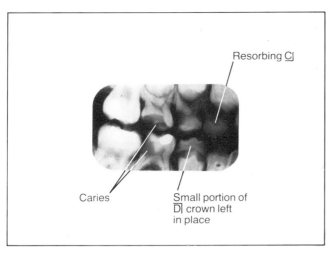

Figure 237. *Right bitewing radiograph of a girl aged 9 years showing almost complete resorption of $\overline{D|}$ crown prior to exfoliation. Gross caries $\dfrac{ED|}{E|}$ is also evident.*

Caries in the crown, particularly when the pulp chamber becomes involved, may result in retention of the roots of the primary molar with the permanent molar erupting between them (Figure 239). Years later the primary tooth roots may still be evident on the radiographs.

In the congenital absence of permanent successors, roots of the primary molars may (Figure 240a), or may not (Figure 240b) resorb. Eventually the tooth may be shed much later in life after very slow radicular resorption.

Figure 238. *Left and right bitewings of a boy aged 8 years showing resorption of mesial aspects of anterior roots of $\overline{D|D}$. This is certainly caused by erupting $\overline{3|3}$.*

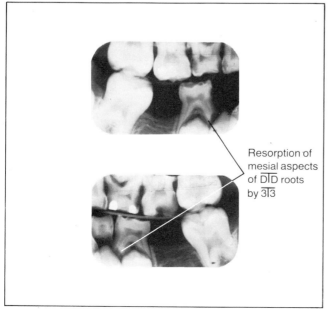

Resorption of mesial aspects of $\overline{D|D}$ roots by $\overline{3|3}$

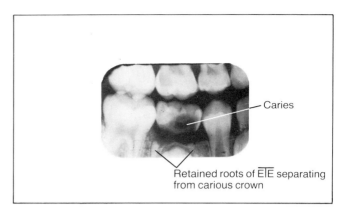

Caries

Retained roots of $\overline{E|E}$ separating from carious crown

Figure 239. *Right bitewing of a girl aged 10 years showing caries separating crown and roots of $\overline{E|}$. $\overline{5|}$ is erupting between the roots, and in such circumstances the roots may remain present for many years without resorption.*

Resorption of Teeth by Abnormal Conditions

External Resorption

Apical infection is a frequent cause of external resorption of roots of both primary (Figure 241a) and permanent (Figure 241b) teeth, and the resorption generally has an area of associated radiolucency. Sclerosis, as in Figure 241b, may surround the radiolucency, and in other instances there may be just sclerosis surrounding the resorbed apex. Figure 241c shows such an appearance on the mesial root of $\overline{6|}$.

Figure 240 (a). *Right bitewing radiograph of a girl aged 15 years showing complete resorption of $\overline{E|}$ roots in the absence of $\overline{5|}$.* (b) *Periapical radiograph of a man aged 21 years showing only slight resorption of $\overline{E|}$ in the absence of $\overline{5|}$.*

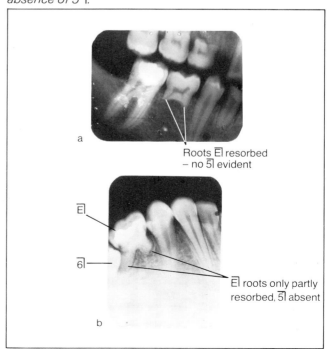

a

Roots $\overline{E|}$ resorbed – no $\overline{5|}$ evident

$\overline{E|}$

$\overline{6|}$

$\overline{E|}$ roots only partly resorbed. $\overline{5|}$ absent

b

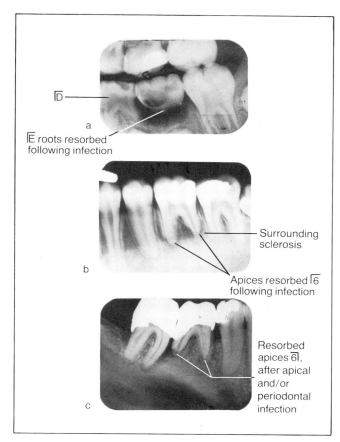

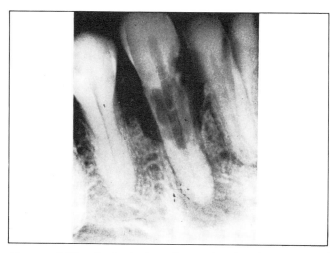

Figure 242. *Periapical radiograph showing external root resorption in* 3⌐ *of a man aged 62 years. The outline of the pulp is preserved which indicates that the resorption has not originated here. The pulp was finally exposed and died resulting in the apical bone change seen here. There is no lamina at the apex.*

D⌐ ——

a

⌐E roots resorbed
following infection

Surrounding
sclerosis

Apices resorbed ⌐6
following infection

b

Resorbed
apices 6⌐,
after apical
and/or
periodontal
infection

c

Figure 241 (a). *Left bitewing radiograph of a child aged 6 years showing complete resorption of* ⌐E *roots following infection arising after carious exposure of the pulp.* (b) *Uneven resorption of the apices of* ⌐6 *seen on the periapical radiograph of a boy aged 18 years. Apical infection following death of the pulp was the cause.* (c) *Periapical radiograph of* 6⌐ *region showing resorption of the apices of* 6⌐ —*probably as the result of death of the pulp and apical infection. The distal root is also involved in local periodontal disease and bone loss — or is this tooth a retained* E⌐?

Periodontal disease may stimulate external resorption. Figure 242 illustrates the lower right canine in a man aged 62 years. Resorption had started mesially in a pocket and extended across the root surface downwards with irregular resorption of the root. The outline of the pulp canal is maintained which enables a differential diagnosis to be made with internal resorption. The pulp had become involved by eventual exposure near the neck of the tooth, and apical infection is evident. There is some bone loss at the neck of the tooth.

Pressure is a frequent cause of resorption. Figure 243 shows resorption of $\frac{51|1}{|1|}$ apices, as a result of pressure from a fixed orthodontic appliance in a boy aged 11 years. The forces used were normal yet the resorption is marked.

In Figure 80 pressure from impacted 8⌐ has resorbed a great deal of 7⌐'s roots, and in Figure 152 unerupted 3⌐

has caused marked resorption of 2⌐ root. Intraoral views are invaluable in showing such conditions and enable an accurate assessment to be made.

Cysts and tumours (Figures 278 and 307) often cause the external resorption of fully-formed roots, or interfere with forming roots (Figure 287f). The lamina dura will reform at the resorbed area when the cause is removed.

Fibrous dysplasia can cause root resorption, and in Figure 244, a case involving a 23 year old woman, roots of 87⌐ have undergone partial resorption. This is hard to see on the radiograph due to the opaque shadow of the thickened bone. A recent socket of 5⌐ is evident. Paget's disease is also known to be associated with resorption, though hypercementosis is more usual.

Trauma is often the cause of resorption and a study of Figures 141 and 142 will show the slight changes in 1|1 following an accident which avulsed |1 and traumatised 1⌐. A more extensive resorption is seen in Figure 245 following replantation of 1⌐ in a girl aged 19 years. The root space has been replaced by bone and the pulps of 21|1 have calcified.

Transplantation of a tooth from one part of the mouth to another may result in a mild or extensive resorption of the root substance (Figure 96), and may be followed by ankylosis. The reason for this resorption is not always obvious.

Submerged teeth not directly associated with the pressures of impactions, cysts or tumours, may undergo partial resorption of roots and crowns (Figure 79). In some instances this resorption may proceed until the original outline of the tooth is hardly evident. On other occasions there is no resorption of buried teeth.

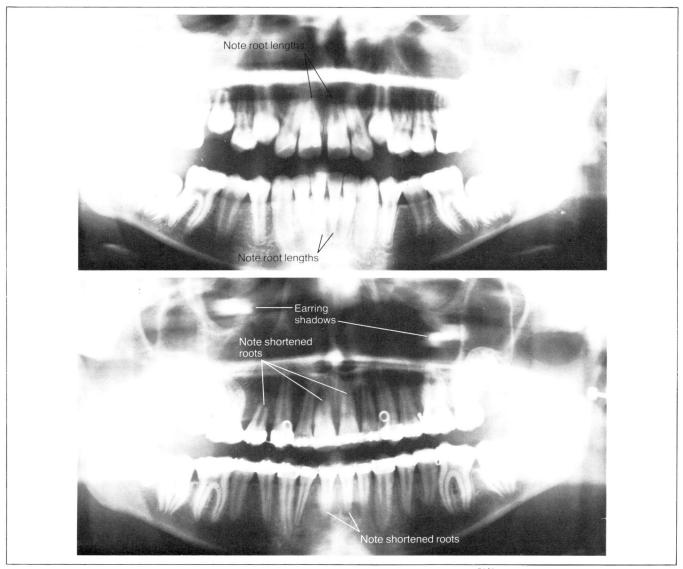

Figure 243. Panelipse radiographs of a boy aged 11 years showing the length of $\frac{5\,1|1}{1|1}$ before **(a)**, and after **(b)**, fixed appliance therapy. The pressure from the appliance has resulted in resorption of the apices of the incisors. It is difficult to say what has happened to the apex of $5|$ as it was incomplete on the first film, but the root is very short and appears to be resorbed. Lamina covers the root ends of these teeth which were all vital.

Figure 244. Periapical radiograph of a woman aged 23 years with fibrous dysplasia of the right maxillary tuberosity and some resorption of $87|$ roots. This is not easy to discern through the thickened bone.

Figure 245. Periapical radiograph of a girl aged 19 years showing complete resorption of $1|$ root, and calcification of pulps in $21|1$. These three teeth had been traumatised, $1|$ having been avulsed and replanted soon afterwards.

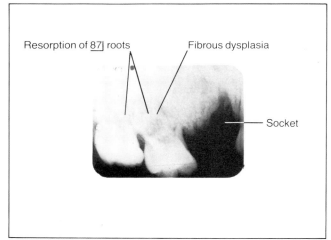

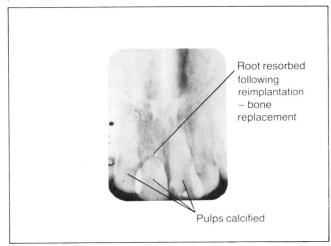

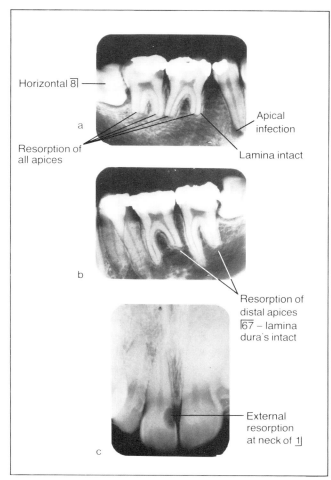

Figure 246 (a). *Periapical radiograph* $\overline{76}$⌉ *region of a woman aged 25 years showing resorption of* $\overline{76}$⌉ *apices, and infection at the apex of the premolar. The lamina is intact across the resorbed apices and there is no suggestion of infection. There was no history of trauma. This is idiopathic resorption.* (b) *Periapical radiograph of the same patient as (a) showing only resorption of the distal apices of* ⌈$\overline{67}$ *with the lamina dura still intact.* (c) *Idiopathic resorption at the neck of* 1⌉ *seen on a periapical radiograph. This could be mistaken for a prepared cavity but it is too sharply outlined for caries.*

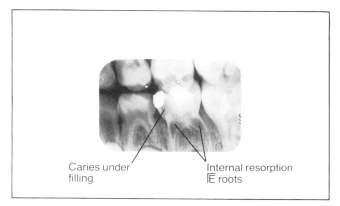

Figure 247. *Left bitewing radiograph of a boy aged 7 years showing internal resorption of the pulp canals in* ⌈E. *The smooth enlargement and loss of the old pulp canal outline are significant features in internal resorption. There is deep mesial caries in this tooth which is almost certainly the cause of the resorption.*

Idiopathic Resorption

Occasionally idiopathic resorption occurs to the roots of teeth (Figure 246a and b). Although the molars are heavily filled it is hard to understand why $\overline{76}$⌉ have had partial resorption of both roots. ⌈$\overline{67}$ have had distal root resorption only. The pulps of all these teeth remain wide up to the resorbed edge with no sign of the characteristic narrowing that occurs towards normal apices (for example mesial roots ⌈$\overline{67}$). In addition the lamina dura is intact on all these teeth.

Idiopathic resorption at the neck of a tooth can be seen in Figure 246c. There was no history of periodontal disease in this patient, and on careful investigation the radiolucent area in 1⌉ crown mesially was found to have a hard wall and no caries. Generally carious cavities will show a more diffuse radiolucent outline than those produced by resorption.

Differential diagnosis of external apical root resorption will have to consider: abnormally short roots; incompletely-formed roots; apicectomied roots; stunted roots from radiation; dilacerated roots; and probably the most common occurrence—foreshortening of the image by radiographic projection. Another factor that must be considered is loss of the lamina around the root making the root appear thinner, so possibly resorbed.

Internal Resorption

Internal, or central resorption as it is sometimes termed, can arise in the primary or permanent dentition, generally as the result of irritation, pulpitis, or infection. The resorption is characterised by widening and loss of the original outline of the root canal. This serves to differentiate internal resorption from external resorption. In the latter the original outline of the pulp canal is retained through the radiolucency of the external resorption.

Figure 247 illustrates internal resorption of the pulp canals in ⌈E. The large carious cavity evident mesially is the likely cause of the condition in this 7 year old boy.

Whereas external resorption frequently presents an irregular pattern, internal resorption generally presents as an expanded smooth-walled radiolucency of the pulp canal (Figures 247, 248 and 249). Unless extensive, these areas seldom communicate with the outside of the tooth root, though by the time they reach the proportion seen in Figure 249 this must be a possibility. It is more likely that the internal resorption in this case arose due to the depth of the filling in ⌊2 than as a result of the close proximity of unerupted ⌈3.

Root canal treatment may prevent further internal resorption, but there is little that can be done to solve external resorption short of extraction—or filling when at the neck of the tooth (Figure 250).

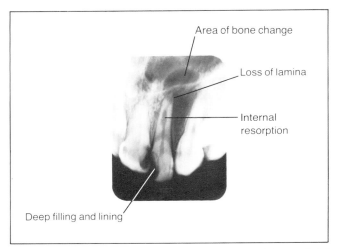

Area of bone change

Loss of lamina

Internal resorption

Deep filling and lining

Figure 248. *Periapical radiograph of a girl aged 16 years showing internal resorption of ⌊2, with widening of the pulp canal outline. There is a very deep mesial filling in this tooth, and a radiolucent area of bone change at the apex which appears cyst-like. Early distal caries is also evident.*

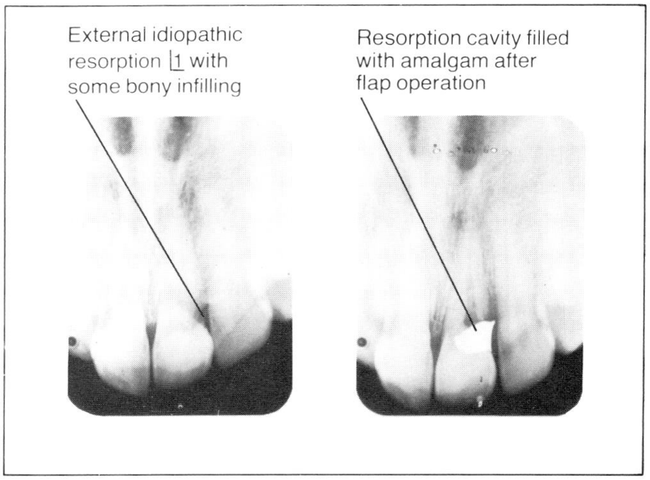

External idiopathic resorption ⌊1 with some bony infilling

Resorption cavity filled with amalgam after flap operation

Figure 250. *Periapical radiographs of a woman aged 50 years. The first radiograph shows idiopathic external resorption at the neck of ⌊1 distally which has been partly infilled with bone. This fact was established clinically when a flap was raised, the resorbed area cleared of bone, and the resulting cavity filled with amalgam.*

Root Canal Treatment

General Considerations

Radiography plays a very important part in endodontics, helping both in the assessment of cases for suitability for root treatment and in depicting the results, satisfactory or otherwise, of manipulative procedures.

It is necessary for the operator to know the length, width and regularity of the pulp canal; whether roots are straight or bent; whether or not calcifications of the pulp are present; and whether or not the pulp canal divides. He also requires to know whether or not his instruments or root filling materials have reached the apex; are short of the apex; have perforated the apex; have perforated the side of the root; or have perforated the bifurcation rather than passed down the canal.

All these factors can be assessed from radiographs provided that a good technique is used.

Figure 249. *Periapical radiograph of a girl aged 18 years with internal resorption of ⌊2, a heavy distal filling, and a closely related ⌊3. ⌊C is retained. In spite of the close relationship with ⌊3 this is a case of internal resorption — probably arising from irritation produced by the filling. The apex of ⌊2 is not visible. As in nearly all cases of internal resorption the original outline of the pulp wall has been lost.*

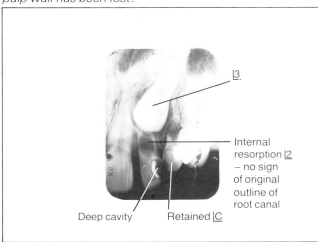

⌊3.

Internal resorption ⌊2 – no sign of original outline of root canal

Deep cavity   Retained ⌊C

Figure 251. *Foreshortened and elongated views of 1⌈1 both taken with the bisected-angle technique within a short period of time. The area of bone change at the apices appears somewhat smaller in the first radiograph than in the second. This is caused by the variation in tube angulation between the two films; the area could not have changed in size between the two radiographs.*

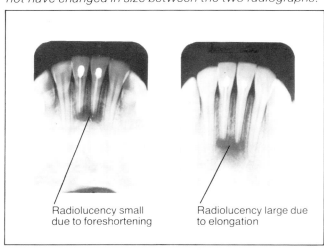

Radiolucency small due to foreshortening

Radiolucency large due to elongation

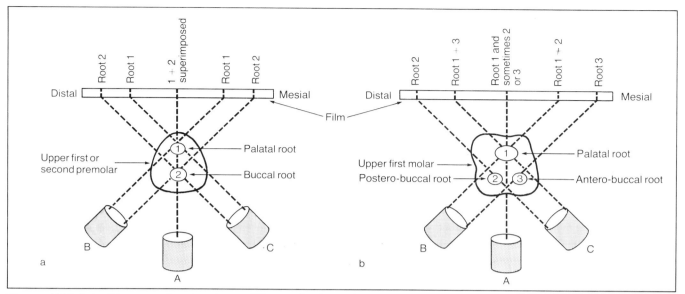

Figure 252 (a). *Diagram showing how different horizontal angulations of the tubehead to the film will assist in showing two root canals in radiographs of upper premolars. With the tubehead at position 'A', palatal root 1 and buccal root 2, will be superimposed on the radiograph. If the tubehead is angulated forwards slightly (position 'B') the palatal root will be projected more distally than the buccal root on the radiograph, hence both will be seen. If the tubehead is angulated backwards slightly (position 'C') the palatal root will be projected more mesially than the buccal root on the radiograph, hence again both will be seen. If the operator notes which of the two angulations he has used he can determine which root is which on the radiograph.* **(b)** *Diagram showing how different horizontal angulations of the tubehead to the film will assist in showing three root canals in radiographs of upper molars. With the tubehead at position 'A' it is generally possible to see the palatal apex of a 3-rooted upper molar. Sometimes one or other of the buccal apices will be superimposed on the palatal root. If the tubehead is moved to position 'B', the antero-buccal root apex will be projected more mesially on the radiograph than the palatal and disto-buccal roots. If the tubehead is moved to position 'C', the disto-buccal root apex will be projected more distally than the palatal and antero-buccal roots. Using this technique it is often possible to separate the roots of 3-rooted teeth on radiographs and determine which is which.*

In most instances the paralleling technique using intraoral film will provide the best radiographic view for endodontics, but carefully positioned bisected angle views are adequate. The latter technique can cause problems in interpreting healing of apical lesions as can be seen in Figure 251. The two radiographic views were taken within a very short period of time yet the area of radiolucency appears much larger in the second film due to elongation of the image.

It may be necessary to vary the horizontal angle of the tubehead to show multi-rooted tooth canals without superimposition of buccal and palatal canals, and Figure 252a and b shows how this is accomplished.

Measuring the Length of Root Canals

Depending on the angles of projection, canals in the bisected angle technique radiograph may appear longer or shorter than they actually are. In the paralleling technique radiograph they will be longer. Figure 253 shows how the true length of the pulp canal can be found. It is then possible to ream the canal without perforating the apex.

Figure 253a represents a radiograph of ⌐1 with a reamer in the pulp canal short of the apex. There is a

'stop' at the neck of the reamer to prevent it perforating the apex. The radiographic image of the reamer, 'stop' to tip, is measured, as is the image of the length of the tooth. The true length of the reamer 'stop' to tip is known (Figure 253b), though the true length of the tooth is not known.

From the formula:

$$\text{True tooth length} = \frac{\text{True reamer length} \times \text{Radiographic tooth length}}{\text{Radiographic reamer length}}$$

we can find the length of reamer required to reach the tooth apex without perforation (Figure 253c and d).

Radiographic Appearance of Different Root Filling Materials

The opacity of root fillings on radiographs can give some indications as to the material used. Polyantibiotic pastes cast no shadows. The opacity of N2 material is seen in Figure 254a, and is similar to the opacity resulting from the use of zinc oxide as a root filling material. GP points cast a slightly more opaque shadow (Figure 254b), as does zinc oxyphosphate cement. Silver points cast a very opaque shadow and are unlikely to be mistaken for other materials (Figure 254c).

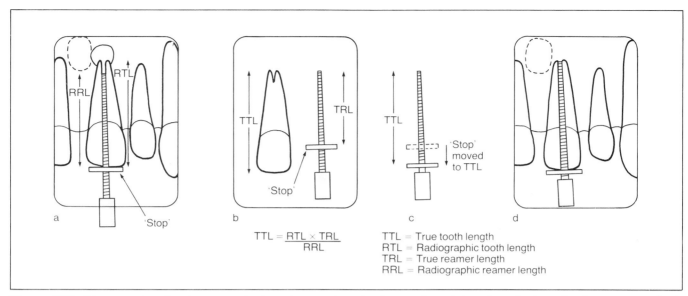

Figure 253. *Diagram showing how to calculate the true length of a tooth and therefore the length of reamer required to exactly reach the apex.* **(a)** *Diagram of radiograph with reamer reaching into apical ⅓ of pulp canal in ⌊1. RTL = radiographic tooth length, RRL = radiographic reamer length.* **(b)** *Diagram of tooth and reamer shows: TTL = true tooth length, TRL = true reamer length. We find the true tooth length from:*

$$TTL = \frac{RTL \times TRL}{RRL}$$

(c) *Having calculated the true tooth length (TTL), the 'stop' is adjusted on the reamer until the true tooth length is the same as the distance from the 'stop' to the reamer tip.* **(d)** *The tooth can then be reamed accurately to the apex without perforation. This is most helpful when treating children's teeth with wide-open apices or incomplete roots.*

Root Fillings in Single-rooted Teeth

Figure 255a to f shows a series of radiographs taken during the root canal treatment of ⌊2 in a boy aged 18 years. The first radiograph (Figure 255a) shows a deep unlined cavity in ⌊2. There is no suggestion of periapical change in this tooth. Six months later (Figure 255b)

Figure 254 (a). *N2 filling material in canals and pulp chamber of 7⌋.* **(b)** *GP point in pulp canal ⌊1. (Note dilacerated ⌊2.)* **(c)** *Silver point in pulp canal ⌊1.*

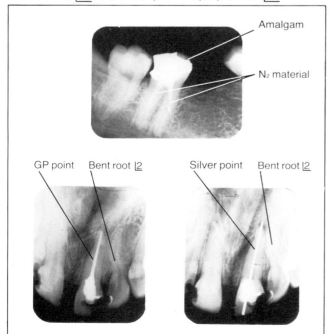

there is an area of radiolucency at the apex of ⌊2 and the tooth is dead. It is evident from the radiograph that the root canal is straight mesio-distally, and wide enough for instrumentation. There are no obvious calcifications of the pulp. The third radiograph (Figure 255c) shows a diagnostic wire in the pulp canal for measurement purposes. The fourth radiograph (Figure 255d) shows that the tooth has been root filled (with GP point and paste), and that some of the material has passed through the apical foramen into the area of radiolucency. Two months later (Figure 255e), the extra paste has been resorbed and the radiolucent area is beginning to decrease in size. After a further 18 months (Figure 255f) the radiolucent area has been filled in with new bone.

Interestingly there has been further resorption of the root filling paste, this time from within the pulp canal. The end of the non-absorbable GP point can now be seen.

This series shows the advantage of radiographs as a diagnostic aid throughout root canal treatment procedures.

Root Filling Multi-rooted Teeth

Two-rooted teeth, e.g. upper first premolars and occasionally the second premolars, are often involved in root canal treatment procedures. Figure 256a to e illustrates the root canal treatment of ⌊5 in a woman aged 20 years. Figure 256a is a bisected angle view of ⌊5 taken with the central ray projected perpendicularly through the contact point to the film. There is a diagnostic wire in the tooth; but it is not evident radiographically that a second canal is present.

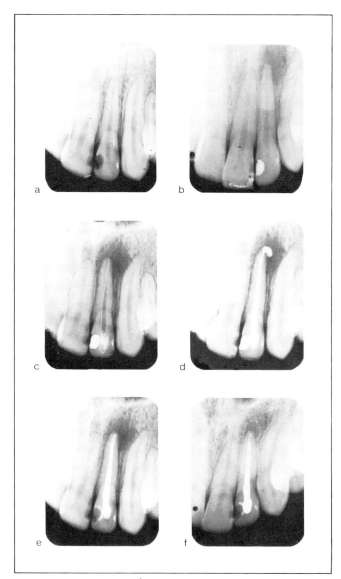

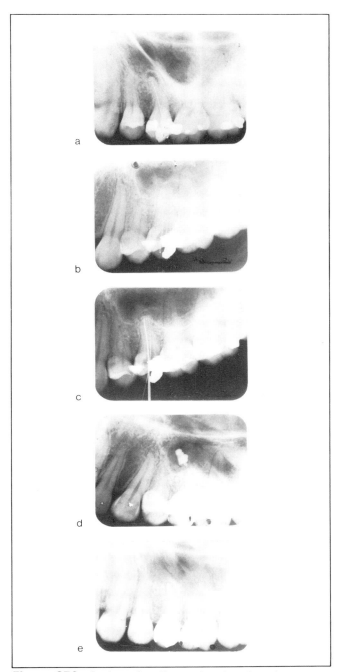

Figure 255 (a). *Apex $\lfloor 2$ appears sound in this boy aged 18 years.* **(b)** *6 months later there is a radiolucent area of bone change at the apex of $\lfloor 2$, with loss of lamina.* **(c)** *Diagnostic wire at the apex of $\lfloor 2$.* **(d)** *Root filling paste through the apex $\lfloor 2$ and GP point within the canal.* **(e)** *2 months after (d) the paste has been absorbed outside the root and the bone is regenerating in the area of radiolucency.* **(f)** *18 months after (e) there has been further resorption of the paste, this time from within the canal at the apex, and there has been further infilling of the radiolucent area with bone. The end of the GP point can now be seen inside the canal.*

Using the technique shown in Figure 252a the operator has projected the central ray slightly more distally in Figure 256b, and both canals can now be seen with diagnostic wires enclosed. The palatal wire does not reach the apex. In the next view (Figure 256c) a narrow reamer does reach the apex in the palatal canal. It is shown that this is the palatal canal from the backward angulation of the central ray (ray 'C' in Figure 252a), and also because the palatal cusp is higher on the radiograph than the buccal cusp in the bisecting angle technique. Figure 256d, a very foreshortened view, shows both canals of $\lfloor 5$ filled and some paste through

Figure 256. *Series of radiographs showing the stages in the root treatment of $\lfloor 5$. Relate these radiographic views to Figure 252(a).* **(a)** *With the central ray at right angles to the film only one canal can be seen in $\lfloor 5$. Area of bone change at the apex is readily visible.* **(b)** *With the horizontal angle changed so that the central ray is projected more distally both canals can be seen. It is also evident that the diagnostic wire in the palatal canal does not reach the apex.* **(c)** *Diagnostic reamer in the palatal canal and diagnostic wire in the buccal canal now reach the apices of $\lfloor 5$.* **(d)** *Both canals of $\lfloor 5$ have been filled and some paste has passed through one or other of the apices — possibly into the antrum or under the mucosal lining.* **(e)** *6 months later the paste outside the root canals has been absorbed.*

the apex. Six months later (Figure 256e) the paste has been absorbed. The radiograph has been taken with a ray perpendicular to the film, and as a result the root-filled canals are superimposed.

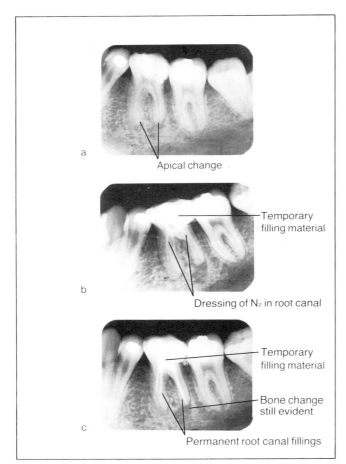

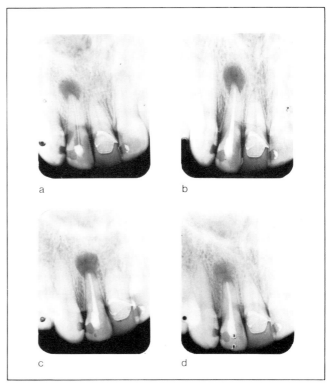

Figure 257 (a). *Periapical radiograph of a boy aged 17 years showing areas of bone change at the apices* $\overline{6}$. **(b)** *N2 dressings in the pulp chamber and root canals of* $\overline{6}$. **(c)** *Root canals of* $\overline{6}$ *filled with N2 material. A further radiograph will be required after some months to check for healing at the apices.*

Figure 257a, b and c show apical infection of $\overline{6}$, semi-opaque dressings in the pulp chambers and canals, and the final root filling. A further follow-up radio-

Figure 258. *Periapical radiograph of* $76\rfloor$ *region in a woman aged 42 years. Three roots of* $7\rfloor$ *have been filled, though these root fillings do not quite reach the apices.* $6\rfloor$ *has also been root treated, but the antero-buccal root has a calcified pulp and shows a residual area of bone change.*

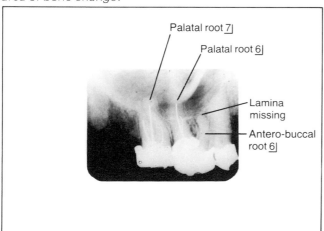

Figure 259 (a). *Periapical radiograph of a woman aged 26 years with a radiolucent area at the apex of* $2\rfloor$ *resembling a granuloma or small cyst. A diagnostic wire is in the pulp canal and reaches almost to the apex.* **(b)** *The root canal has been filled to the apex of* $2\rfloor$. **(c)** *The apical tip of* $2\rfloor$ *has been removed, and the radiolucent area curetted to remove what turned out to be a granuloma.* **(d)** *3 months later healing has taken place and bone has formed across the apex.*

graph is necessary to ensure that the treatment has been successful.

Figure 258 shows completed root treatment of $76\rfloor$ in a woman aged 42 years. There is little sign of an antero-buccal root canal in $6\rfloor$, though the root is readily evident.

Root Canal Filling and Apicectomy

Figure 259a, b, c and d show the stages in the root canal treatment of $2\rfloor$ with a small granuloma at the apex. The diagnostic wire in Figure 259a reaches the apex and following the root canal filling an apicectomy was performed to eradicate the granuloma (Figure 259c). Three months later (Figure 259d) bone is filling in the area above the resected root end.

A much larger area of bone change is seen in the series of radiographs shown in Figure 260. Figure 260a shows areas of periapical change on $\lfloor12$, the area on $\lfloor2$ being of considerable size. GP points were inserted into the canals following cleansing procedures, and Figure 260b shows them extending through the apices into the radiolucent areas.

Apicectomy was performed and a large amount of root was removed from both teeth (Figure 260c). Pieces of GP can be seen at the apices reminiscent of retro-

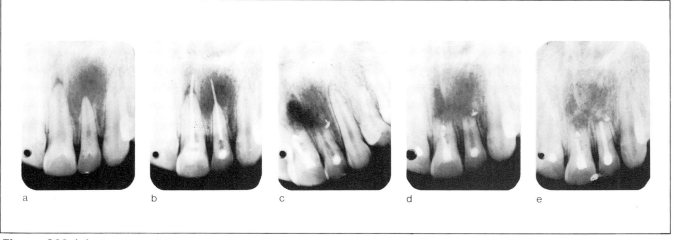

a   b   c   d   e

Figure 260 (a). *Large radiolucent area at the apex of ⌊2, and small area at the apex of ⌊1 overlying the anterior palatine canal in this girl aged 19 years.* **(b)** *GP points well through the apices of ⌊12.* **(c)** *Apicectomied ⌊12, both having lost rather a lot of root. What look like retrograde root fillings are near the apices, but these are probably bits of gutta percha debris. The GP point has been dislodged from the canal of ⌊2 during the operation.* **(d)** *4 months later there has been complete infilling of the radiolucent cavity by bone.* **(e)** *6 months later, a new GP point has been placed in ⌊2.*

grade plugs. Their opacity appears less than that produced by amalgam. The GP point has been lost from ⌊2 during the operation, and that in ⌊1 does not fill the width of the canal. Some healing of the radiolucent area with infilling of bone is evident in Figure 260d, and six months later, Figure 260e, a new GP point has been placed in ⌊2 and further bone organisation has taken place.

Sometimes bone fails to regenerate following apicectomy and there may be sinus formation evident clinically and a discrete area of bone deficiency radiographically. Figure 261 shows such an appearance six months after apicectomy.

Root Filling of Fractured Teeth

It is sometimes necessary to attempt root treatment of fractured teeth when the coronal pulp dies—Figure 262 illustrates such a condition. In this case it was not possible to get the reamer through into the detached apex due to displacement of the latter, so the root filling was taken to the point of fracture. There was no further trouble from the tooth.

Trauma in root canal therapy is covered in Chapter 4.

Lateral Canals and Retrograde Root Fillings

Root treatment of lateral or secondary canals is not simple, but if the area of infection does arise from these some attempt can be made to save the tooth. Figure 263 shows the stages in the root treatment of ⌊1 with infection arising from a lateral canal. Extensive apical resection was not indicated as the tooth appeared to have a very short root. Minimal root resection was performed, and at the same time a lateral retrograde root filling in amalgam was placed in the secondary canal. In the last radiograph of the series (Figure 263e) healing is evident.

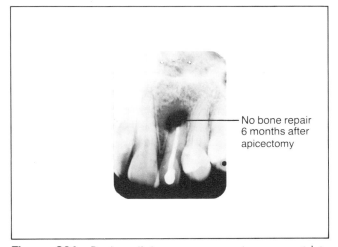

No bone repair 6 months after apicectomy

Figure 261. *Dark radiolucent area at the apex of ⌊2, six months after apicectomy. Clinically there was some suppuration from a sinus in the scar tissue. This is the appearance when bone healing has not taken place.*

Figure 262. *Periapical radiograph showing root filling in the coronal part of fractured 1⌋. The apical fragment is quite healthy.*

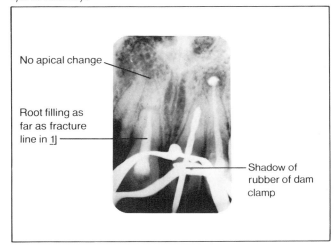

No apical change

Root filling as far as fracture line in 1⌋

Shadow of rubber of dam clamp

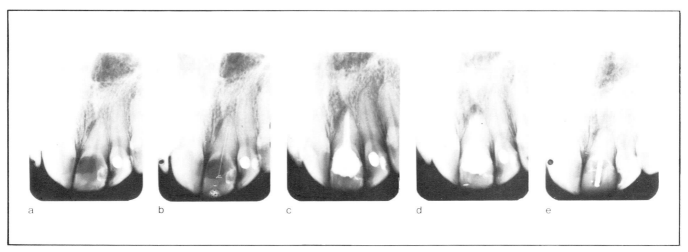

Figure 263. *Series of periapical radiographs of a woman aged 24 years with an area of bone change on a lateral pulp canal in ⌊1. **(a)** Small area of bone change mesially near the apex of ⌊1. **(b)** Diagnostic wire reaching almost to the apex of ⌊1. **(c)** Root filling to apex of ⌊1, area mesially still evident. **(d)** Appearance following apicectomy of apical tip ⌊1 and retrograde root filling on the mesial aspect of the root at the secondary canal. **(e)** 7 months later there has been bone repair at the apex and mesial aspect of ⌊1, but lamina has not yet reformed across the lateral retrograde amalgam root filling.*

Examples of the radiographic appearance of apical retrograde root fillings with amalgam are seen in Figures 142 and 147.

Figure 264. *Three stages in the attempt to save ⌈6 in a woman aged 29 years. To clear the infection at the bifurcation resulting from periodontal disease the mesial root has been resected. The distal root has been retained and root filled to the apex.*

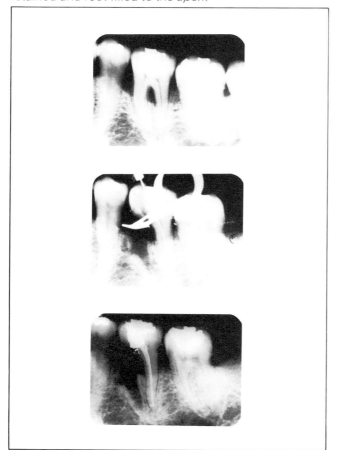

Surgical Removal of One Root in Molars

Lower molars often have bifurcation involvement in periodontal disease. Sometimes it is decided to treat one root and remove the other. The same procedure can be used when one apex fails to heal following root treatment. Figure 264 illustrates a typical case, the mesial root of ⌈6 being removed to help clear infection at the bifurcation and the distal root being retained by root treatment.

Difficult Teeth

Dilacerated teeth (Figure 254b), and dilated odontomes do not lend themselves readily to root treatment. Bent or hooked roots (Figure 265), and split pulps in single-rooted teeth (Figures 243 and 266) make root canal treatment very difficult. Blockage of canals by instru-

Figure 265. *Very thin or calcified pulp is evident in anterior root of 6⌉. Although attempts have been made it has not been possible to get root treatment instruments into this root which is also bent at the apex.*

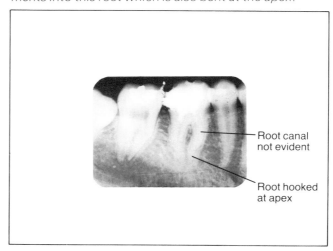

Root canal not evident

Root hooked at apex

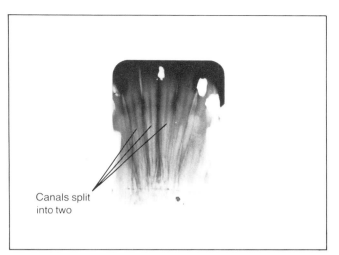

Canals split
into two

Figure 266. *Split pulps in lower anteriors. This elongated radiographic view shows why root canal treatment would be very difficult to perform in the apical part of such teeth. The instrument would generally only reach the point at which the canal divides.*

ments, pulp stones or dentine bridges can make root treatment impossible and it may be necessary in such cases to resort to retrograde root fillings.

Figure 267. *Periapical radiographic series over a period of 2 years in a girl following vital pulpotomy to 1|1.* **(a)** *Fracture of mesial incisal angles of 1|1, apices incomplete.* **(b)** *Pulp chambers have been cleaned out and dressings of calcium hydroxide (not visible on the radiograph) inserted and covered with zinc oxyphosphate cement. The apices are still incomplete.* **(c)** *Four months later thick dentine bridges have formed across the pulp canal but the roots are still incomplete.* **(d)** *One year later the dentine bridges are well shown and the roots of 1|1 are now complete.* **(e)** *One year later still the apices of 1|1 have closed.*

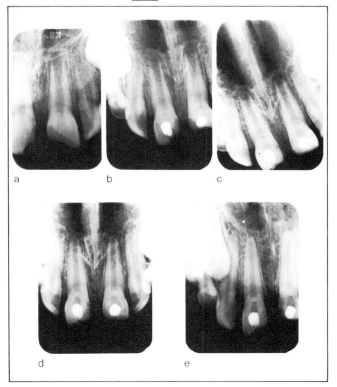

Endodontics in Children

Root treatment of both primary and permanent teeth is undertaken in children, and early damage of the permanent incisors can cause problems as often the roots are incomplete or the apices wide open.

Pulpotomy

If pulps are exposed by trauma, vital pulpotomy may be considered. By placing a dressing of calcium hydroxide in the pulp chamber it is hoped that a dentine bridge will be laid down across the pulp and that the root apex will continue to develop and close (see Figure 267).

Figure 268. *Periapical radiographic series over a period of 4 years in a boy aged 8 years following trauma to 1|1.* **(a)** *|1 has been intruded and the edge fractured, and 1| has been slightly extruded. Apices of 1|1 are wide open and the roots are incomplete.* **(b)** *One year after filling with calcium hydroxide there is no sign of further root development of |1. 1| has had further trauma with near exposure of the pulp. Roots of 1|2 are almost complete.* **(c)** *One year later the roots of 21|1 are complete but there appears to be no change at the apex of |1. With care it can be seen that the end of |1 root does appear to be closing across a little. Clinically there was an obstruction to instrumentation near the apex.* **(d)** *Root filling with GP points and zinc oxide has been completed and there is no sign of periapical infection. Clinically there was a calcific barrier at the apex. Apices of 1|2 have closed. 18 months after this radiograph was taken the patient again fractured 1| !*

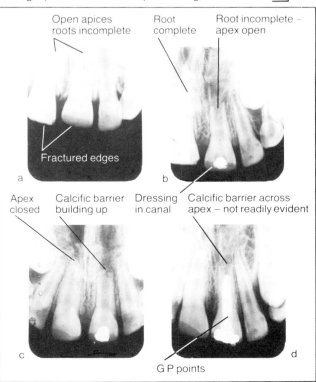

Open apices roots incomplete

Root complete

Root incomplete – apex open

Fractured edges

Apex closed

Calcific barrier building up

Dressing in canal

Calcific barrier across apex – not readily evident

G P points

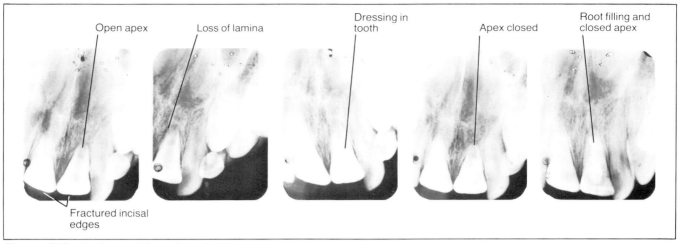

Figure 269. *Radiographic series of a boy aged 10 years showing root treatment to ⌊1 following trauma. All views of 1⌊1 are very foreshortened by the radiographic projection.* **(a)** *Incisal edges of 1⌊1 have been fractured and clinically there was a sinus over ⌊1. The apices are open and the coronal pulp of 1⌋ appears to be calcified.* **(b)** *One month later the lamina and bone have thinned at the apex of ⌊1.* **(c)** *A dressing of calcium hydroxide and barium sulphate has been placed in the root canal and the apex is closing. There is also consolidation of bone at the apex.* **(d)** *Eight months later the apices of 1⌊1 have closed, and the pulp of 1⌋ appears to have calcified.* **(e)** *Eighteen months after (d) the apex of ⌊1 appears to be completely closed, and a satisfactory root canal filling of GP points is in place. The periapical bone appears healthy.*

Induction of Root Completion and Closure

Sometimes a root will fail to develop following trauma, though it is possible that the wide-open apex may be bridged by calcific material following pulp canal cleansing and the insertion of a calcium hydroxide dressing. In Figure 268 the root of ⌊1 in this child aged 8 years, has failed to develop, but a calcific barrier, not readily

evident in the radiograph, has formed across the root end and has enabled root treatment to be completed satisfactorily. The operator could feel a solid end to the canal when inserting the root filling.

In Figure 269 a more definite apical closure can be seen in ⌊1 of this boy aged 10 years. He had sustained incisal edge fracture of 1⌊1 and presented with a sinus

Figure 270. *Radiographic series of a girl aged 8 years showing apical closure of 1⌊1 following trauma.* **(a)** *Trauma to 1⌊1 has caused resorption to the lamina dura surrounding root of ⌊1. The incisal edge has been fractured, the root is not quite complete, and the apex is open.* **(b)** *One year later the roots of 1⌊1 appear complete but the apices are still open. Both teeth gave a positive response to the electric pulp tester, though this result was suspect.* **(c)** *Four months later both teeth were found to be dead and the apices were still open — obviously! Polyantibiotic paste was inserted into the root canals followed two months later by dressings of calcium hydroxide and barium sulphate.* **(d)** *Two years later the apices of 1⌊1 have closed completely. Shortly after this radiograph was taken the teeth were root filled with GP points.* **(e)** *Four years later the apices of 1⌊1 are sound and the periapical bone is healthy.*

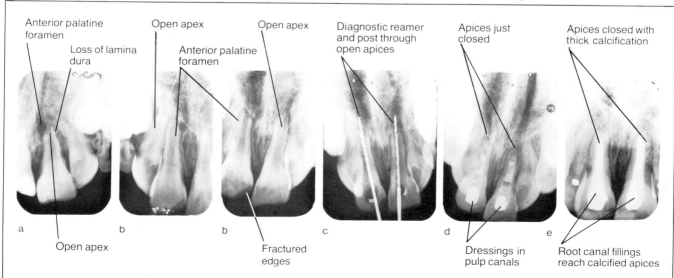

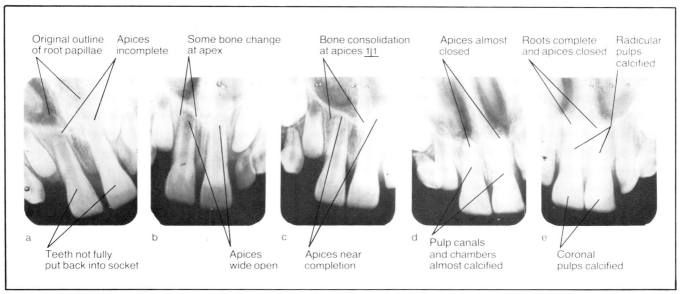

Original outline of root papillae
Apices incomplete
Some bone change at apex
Bone consolidation at apices 1|1
Apices almost closed
Roots complete and apices closed
Radicular pulps calcified

a
b
c
d
e

Teeth not fully put back into socket
Apices wide open
Apices near completion
Pulp canals and chambers almost calcified
Coronal pulps calcified

Figure 271. *Radiographic series of a boy aged 7 years showing completion of roots and calcification of pulps following trauma to 1|1. (a) A local dental surgeon has reimplanted 1| and repositioned |1 following a fairground accident. |1 had been severely displaced. Both teeth have been repositioned with the full clinical crown showing instead of that portion appropriate to his age. The dentine papilla is well separated from the root end. (b) Five months later there has been some consolidation of bone around 1|1. (c) Three months later (b) the root apices are beginning to close. (d) One year after (c) the roots are complete, the apices closed, and the pulps have narrowed markedly. (e) One year after (d) the pulps have calcified, there is lamina dura across the apices, and no sign of periapical infection.*

over |1. This tooth was opened and calcium hydroxide and barium sulphate were placed in the canal. Within 8 months the apex had closed and it was possible to root fill the tooth satisfactorily with GP points.

Incomplete and open apices 1|1 can be seen in a girl aged 8 years in Figure 270. These teeth were pushed back into the maxilla when damaged at the local swimming pool. 1| remained vital, but |1 failed to respond to vitality tests. Eventually both teeth were found to have necrotic pulps and were dressed with polyantibiotic paste (at which point the apices were still open), and later dressed with calcium hydroxide and barium sulphate. At the end of a 2 year period (Figure 270d) the apices had closed and the canals were filled perma-

nently. Four years later (Figure 270e) the apices were sound and the surrounding bone was healing.

There are instances where root canal treatment is unnecessary to save avulsed and seriously displaced teeth (Figure 271). Within an hour of avulsion of 1| and displacement of |1 in this boy aged 7 years a general dental practitioner reimplanted 1| and repositioned |1 splinting the two teeth with self-cure acrylic. This series of radiographs show the changes taking place at the root ends and in the pulp chambers and canals over a period of $2\frac{1}{2}$ years. The apices complete, and the pulp canals narrow until only a thin thread is evident. Eventually even this disappears. There has been no resorption of the roots of either tooth.

7. Cysts of the Jaws

Dental cysts arise as a result of proliferation of epithelial cells. This cell mass liquefies centrally and becomes a cyst, which increases in size by osmosis. Its outline is determined to some extent by the resistance it meets, though it tends to remain circular.

Radiographs are essential to show the extent and shape of these fluid-filled cavities. If untreated, the cyst will eventually destroy the overlying bone and distend the soft tissues. There is then the possibility of pathological fracture.

When dental cysts involve the antral cavity they:

1. Erode the antral floor.
2. Erode the lamina dura and roots of the related teeth.
3. Remove the bone pattern from the antral wall.

These factors help to differentiate between a cyst and the antrum. In addition, the cyst, unless infected, will tend to have a less dense outline.

Cysts are usually discovered as a result of expansion of the jaw, when acute infection supervenes, or as a chance finding during dental radiography.

Radiographic views should be taken to show the full extent of cysts and it is often necessary to have extraoral views. The standard occipitomental view is useful for demonstrating cysts involving the antrum.

Radiographic Appearance of Cyst

The radiographic appearance of cyst is a radiolucent area, tending to be circular in outline (particularly in the early stages), bordered by sometimes normal bone with no apparent cortex; sometimes a definite opaque thin cortical layer; and sometimes, when infection has supervened, an opaque thick diffuse cortical layer.

On occasions there may be calcifications within the cyst. These are often related to supplemental and supernumerary teeth, and odontomes of all types.

Cysts of the maxilla seldom cross the midline until they are very large indeed, except when they are midline fissural cysts, in which case they tend to spread out to both sides from the midline.

A differential diagnosis has to be made with other apical radiolucencies, and this matter has been dealt with in Chapter 5.

A convenient classification of cysts is given in Table 2.

Figure 272. *Periapical radiograph of a man aged 20 years, illustrating what could be either a small cyst or a large area of infection. There is a rounded area of bone destruction between 32 | and at 2 | apex. In addition there is periapical infection at apex 1 | .*

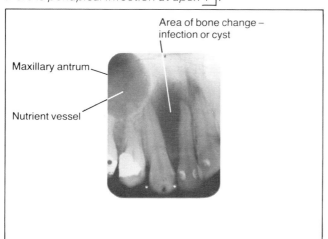

Area of bone change – infection or cyst

Maxillary antrum

Nutrient vessel

Table 2. Classification of cysts.

Odontogenic cysts
Radicular cysts
    Apical dental cyst (periodontal)
    Lateral periodontal cyst
    Residual cyst
Developmental cysts
    Cyst of eruption
    Dentigerous cyst
    Primordial cyst
Cystic neoplasms
    Ameloblastoma

Non-odontogenic cysts
Fissural cysts
    Incisive canal cyst
    Globulomaxillary cyst (doubtful entity)
    Nasolabial cyst
    Median mandibular (and maxillary) cyst
Non-epithelialized bone cysts
Latent bone cyst — Stafne cavity
Antral mucosal retention cysts

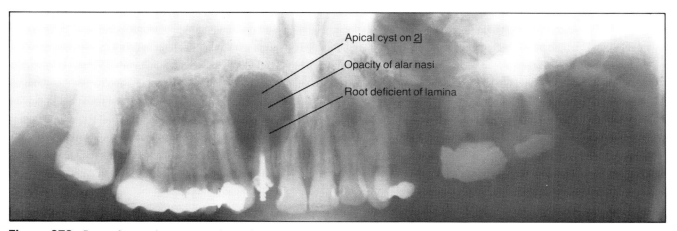

Figure 273. *Part of a static panoramic radiograph of a man aged 29 years showing 2| apex associated with a discrete radiolucent area of bone change extending from 3| to 1| . This is almost certainly an apical cyst on 2| .*

Labels on figure:
Apical cyst on 2|
Opacity of alar nasi
Root deficient of lamina

Odontogenic Cysts

Odontogenic cysts arise from epithelial cells related to dental structures, such as the enamel organ and epithelial debris of Malassez. They are generally lined by stratified squamous epithelium, and if any other lining is present, it may well *not* be an odontogenic cyst that is being considered.

Figure 274 (a). *Periapical radiograph of a woman aged 20 years showing deep invaginated cingulum pit in 2| . There is a large area of radiolucency at the apex of this tooth representative of cyst.* **(b)** *Periapical radiograph of a woman of 31 years showing deep invaginated cingulum pit in 2| . There is a large radiolucent area related to this tooth, which is a likely cyst. 3| root has been displaced distally. The oval radiolucent area above 1| apex is the anterior palatine fossa.*

Radicular (Periodontal) Cysts

Apical Dental Cyst

It is often difficult, if not impossible, to tell the difference between infection, a granuloma and early cyst on a radiograph. Figure 272 could be either a small cyst or a large area of infection. The radiolucent area associated with 2| has no obvious cortex and is rather indefinite. 1| has a small area of bone change at the apex indicative of periapical infection.

Figure 273 is the typical radiographic appearance of dental cyst on root-filled and post-crowned 2| . The radiolucent area is circumscribed, and lamina dura is missing from the apex of 2| . On the original radiograph a lamina can be seen surrounding the 1| root.

Figure 275 (a). *Periapical radiograph of a boy aged 14 years. There is a cyst related to dead |2 which has displaced the roots of |34 distally.* **(b)** *Radiograph of same patient showing that the cyst has not crossed the midline in spite of the displacement of the |34.*

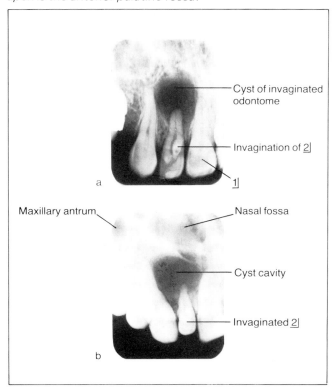

Labels on figure 274:
Cyst of invaginated odontome
Invagination of 2|
1|
Maxillary antrum
Nasal fossa
Cyst cavity
Invaginated 2|
a
b

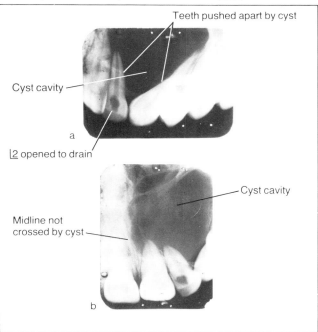

Labels on figure 275:
Teeth pushed apart by cyst
Cyst cavity
|2 opened to drain
a
Cyst cavity
Midline not crossed by cyst
b

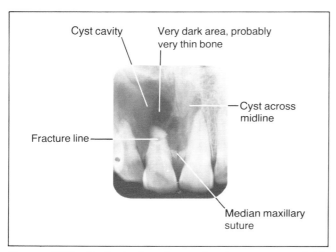

Cyst cavity — Very dark area, probably very thin bone

Cyst across midline

Fracture line

Median maxillary suture

Figure 276. *Periapical radiograph of a man aged 32 years showing radicular periodontal cyst arising on 1⌋ with a fractured root. The cyst has crossed the midline extending from behind ⌊1 almost to 4⌋ (not shown).*

Apical cysts are often associated with invaginated odontomes and teeth with deep cingulum pits (Figure 274a and b).

As apical cysts enlarge, they tend to push the adjacent teeth apart, sometimes markedly so (Figure 275a), yet in the maxilla the cyst will tend not to cross the midline (Figure 275b).

Figure 276 shows a cyst arising on 1⌋ with a fractured root. In this case the cyst *has* crossed the midline and appears to extend behind ⌊1 to the 4⌋ region. No well-defined cortex is evident and there is no marked separation of the roots of the related teeth. The opaque cortical wall of the antrum is in marked contrast to the outline wall of the cyst. Sometimes the wall of a cyst will show the same density and thickness as the wall of the antrum causing some confusion in the differential diagnosis.

Figure 277 shows part of an apical cyst in a woman aged 41 years extending from the midline to 6⌋ region,

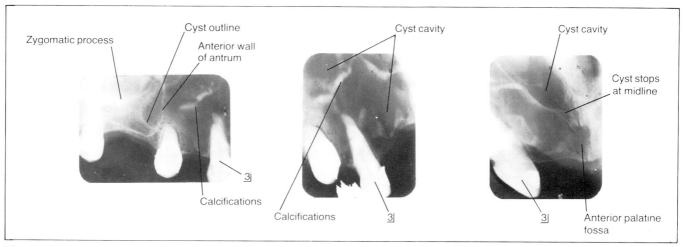

Zygomatic process — Cyst outline — Anterior wall of antrum — Cyst cavity — Cyst cavity — Cyst stops at midline — Calcifications — Calcifications — 3⌋ — 3⌋ — 3⌋ — Anterior palatine fossa

Figure 277. *Periapical radiographs of a woman aged 41 years, the appearance is that of a large dental residual cyst which has not crossed the midline. The cyst cavity contains several patches of calcification and extends from the midline to 6⌋ region, bulging into the antrum.*

Figure 278. *Periapical radiographs of a woman aged 21 years showing large radiolucent cyst-like area extending from 6⌉ to ⌊7 region. There was little clinical evidence of expansion although the cyst extended from the apices of the teeth to the lower border of the mandible with some erosion of the cortex. There is no obvious displacement of the teeth, though there is the suggestion of some resorption of ⌊6 roots. 5⌉5 have been extracted and cyst could have arisen from either of these teeth. Amalgam residue has dropped into 5⌉ socket at the time of extraction.*

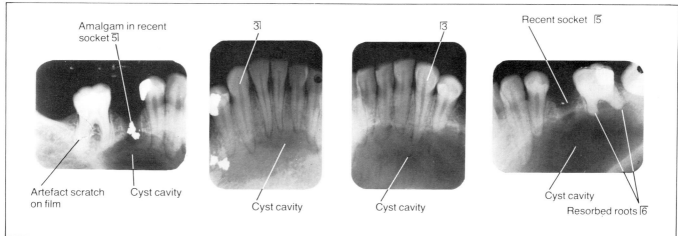

Amalgam in recent socket 5⌉ — 3⌋ — ⌊3 — Recent socket ⌊5

Artefact scratch on film — Cyst cavity — Cyst cavity — Cyst cavity — Cyst cavity — Resorbed roots ⌊6

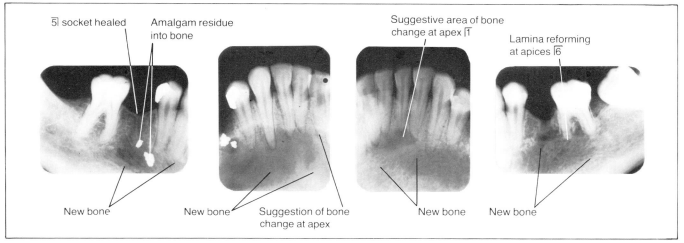

Figure 279. *Periapical radiographs of same patient as Figure 278 two years later. There has been almost complete infilling of the cyst cavity with bone, but ⌐1 has an area of bone change at the apex and is non-vital. This tooth could have been the original cause of the cyst.*

and containing particles of calcification. The radiograph depicts the cyst bulging into the antrum, yet it does not cross the midline.

The cortex of the mandible is very thick and solid presenting a barrier to the expanding cyst. As a result the cyst will sometimes extend a considerable distance along the cancellous bone before expanding the cortex. Figure 278 shows such a case, the cyst extending from 6̄⌐ region to ⌐7 region with resorption only of the roots of ⌐6 which was vital. The cyst was discovered one month after removal of 5̄|5̄ as a result of some swelling in ⌐5 region, and could have arisen from either of these premolar teeth. The cyst was marsupialized and packed, then later a GP bung was retained for nearly six months. Two years later healing was almost complete (Figure 279), but it was noticed that lamina was missing from the apex of ⌐1. The tooth was found to be non-vital and may have been the original cause of the cyst. ⌐1 was root treated and the apical lesion disappeared. Amalgam foreign bodies can be seen on the radiographs which dropped into the socket during the extraction of 5̄|.

Figure 280. *Periapical radiograph of a boy aged 17 years showing |2̄ with root filling and radiolucent area at the apex. The radiograph also shows what transpired to be a lateral periodontal cyst near the neck of |2̄ close to |3̄.*

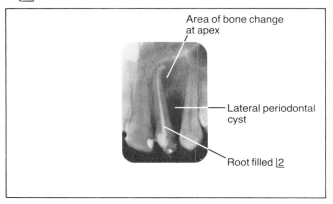

Figure 281. *Periapical and occlusal radiographs of a man aged 43 years showing a large radiolucent area extending from above 4| to 7| region. Roots of 75| are displaced. There is considerable buccal expansion and thinning of the bone. All the teeth were vital suggesting the diagnosis to be residual cyst.*

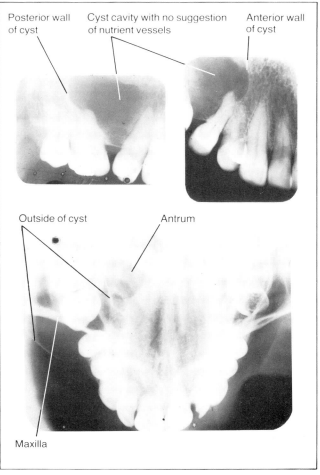

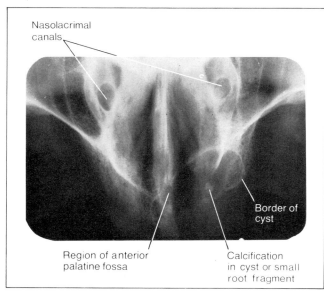

Nasolacrimal canals

Border of cyst

Region of anterior palatine fossa

Calcification in cyst or small root fragment

Figure 282. *Standard occlusal radiograph of a woman aged 67 years showing a large radiolucent area extending from midline to ⌊4 region. There are two opaque fragments evident which could be calcifications. The appearance suggests residual cyst, or just possibly dental cyst on root fragments. The anterior palatine fossa can be seen in the midline merging into the cyst shadow.*

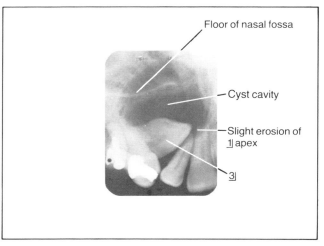

Floor of nasal fossa

Cyst cavity

Slight erosion of 1⌋ apex

3⌋

Figure 283. *Periapical radiograph of a man aged 51 years showing 3⌋ lying obliquely with the crown almost reaching the midline. This is a dentigerous cyst on 3⌋ but 5421⌋ should be tested for vitality.*

secondary root canal in ⌊2. The tooth has an apical area of bone change and has been root treated.

Residual Cyst

There may be a cyst present at the apex of a tooth when the latter is extracted, and it is quite common to note a small granuloma or cyst still attached to the root of the tooth on extraction. Larger cysts will not come away with the tooth but remain behind, the socket healing over and the cyst continuing to expand. This is a residual cyst. Figure 281 shows a standard occlusal radiograph and periapical views of a man aged 43 years with a residual cyst in 6 ⌋region. The roots of vital 75⌋ have been displaced by the cyst, which suggests the diagnosis of cyst, but the standard occlusal view shows the expansion of the maxilla well and leaves no doubt in

Lateral Periodontal Cyst

Lateral periodontal cysts may arise at the side of the root of a tooth due to the irritation or inflammation at the opening of a secondary root canal. It is also possible, if the tooth is vital, that the cyst has arisen as the result of inflammation in a gingival pocket. Figure 280 illustrates lateral periodontal cyst arising between ⌊23 possibly caused by irritation from the pulp of a

Figure 284 (a). *Periapical radiograph of boy aged 10 years, showing root filled 1⌋ and root treatment of ⌊1 which had died following trauma. Crypt of ⌊3 is evident but not overlarge.* **(b)** *Same patient four years later with large radiolucent area associated with unerupted ⌊3. The pulp of ⌊2 has calcified and this tooth may have caused the cyst. However, it is more likely to have arisen from ⌊3 as a dentigerous cyst.*

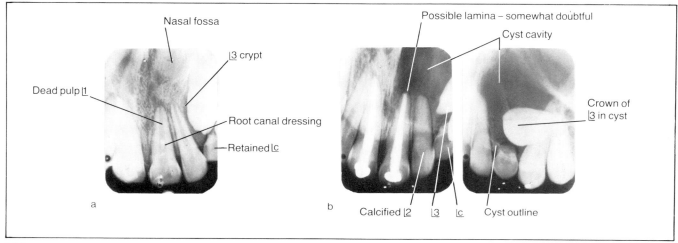

Nasal fossa

⌊3 crypt

Dead pulp ⌊1

Root canal dressing

Retained ⌊c

Possible lamina – somewhat doubtful

Cyst cavity

Crown of ⌊3 in cyst

a

b

Calcified ⌊2   ⌊3   ⌊c   Cyst outline

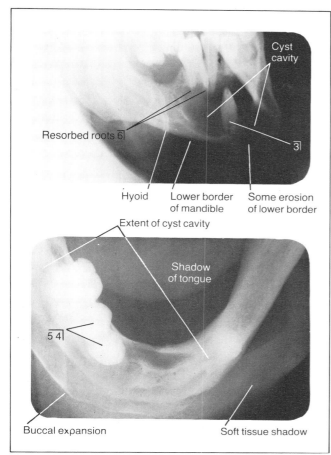

Figure 285 labels:
- Cyst cavity
- Resorbed roots 6⌋
- 3⌋
- Hyoid
- Lower border of mandible
- Some erosion of lower border
- Extent of cyst cavity
- Shadow of tongue
- 5 4⌋
- Buccal expansion
- Soft tissue shadow

Figure 285. *Oblique lateral and occlusal radiographs of a man aged 42 years showing dentigerous cyst on 3⌋, the tooth having been displaced downwards with the long axis still vertical. Thinning of the cortex of the lower border can be seen on the oblique lateral view and the buccal expansion is well shown on the occlusal radiograph.*

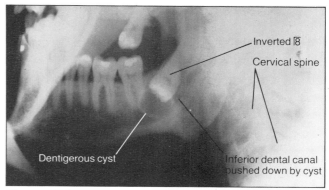

Figure 286 labels:
- Inverted ⌐8
- Cervical spine
- Dentigerous cyst
- Inferior dental canal pushed down by cyst

Figure 286. *Oblique lateral radiograph of a man aged 48 years showing ⌐8 almost inverted with a small dentigerous cyst over and round its crown.*

markedly displaced. Figure 283 depicts a dentigerous cyst on a curved-rooted 3⌋ in a man aged 51 years. Although there is no apparent lamina surrounding 2⌋, this tooth was vital. There appears to be slight erosion of 1⌋.

It can sometimes be difficult to differentiate between dentigerous and apical cysts. Following an accident at 10 years of age 1|1 in the patient shown in Figure 284 died and required root treatment. At this time the apex of ⌊2 appeared normal, as did the crypt of unerupted ⌊3.

Four years later (Figure 284b) there is a large cystic area involving the crown of ⌊3, the pulp of ⌊2 has calcified and the lamina is considerably thinned around this tooth. This is most likely a dentigerous cyst on ⌊3, but it could just possibly have arisen as an apical cyst on ⌊2 and involved ⌊3 later.

Unerupted canines are often involved with dentigerous cysts, and Figure 285 shows a dentigerous cyst on 3⌋ in a man aged 42 years. The buccal expansion can be seen on the true lower occlusal radiograph, though 3⌋ cannot as it is obscured by the opacity of 4⌋.

The lower third molar is commonly related to a dentigerous cyst and Figure 286 shows an inverted ⌐8 with a small dentigerous cyst in a man aged 48 years.

Figure 287a to f illustrates a rather sad tale: Figure 287a and b shows a large dentigerous cyst on the right lower second molar in a boy aged 8 years. The posterior part of the body, the angle and the ramus are considerably expanded. The boy attended with acute infection of the cyst which was treated initially with antibiotics and drainage. A week later the cyst was marsupialized.

Two months after the operation the cyst had shrunk in size taking the developing second molar upwards and inwards (Figure 287c), and there had been thickening of the previously very thin mandibular bone. A further seven months later the tooth was nearly ready to erupt (Figure 287d and e), and the mandible was remodelling well.

the mind that a cyst is present. There is a well marked outline to the cyst which is thinned anteriorly.

Figure 282 shows a residual cyst in ⌊1-4 region with an opaque fragment which could be either calcification within the cyst, or a superimposed odontome.

Developmental Cysts

Cyst of Eruption

Cysts that have formed from the enamel organ in unerupted teeth, and are then destroyed as a result of eruption of the teeth, are termed cysts of eruption. They seldom involve bone to any extent and are recognized clinically rather than radiologically.

Dentigerous Cyst

A dentigerous cyst is one that develops from the enamel organ of an unerupted or impacted tooth which fails to erupt. The crown of the tooth involved generally projects into the cyst cavity, and the tooth itself may be

Three years later (Figure 287f) there had been complete healing of the cyst, but $\overline{7|}$ (note the shape of the roots) had deep mesial caries and had to be extracted. What a waste! In addition, $\overline{5|}$ was impacted and unable to erupt into the arch.

Figure 288 shows a dentigerous cyst on $\overline{8|}$ in a man aged 34 years, where there has been little, if any, displacement of the tooth. The cyst extends downwards and forwards to thin the lower border of the mandible and the occlusal radiograph gives an indication of the buccal bone expansion.

Figure 287 (a). *Posteroanterior radiograph of large dentigerous cyst on the right lower second molar in a boy aged 8 years. The posterior part of the body, the angle and the ramus are markedly expanded. The lesion presented with acute infection which was treated with antibiotics and drainage. A week later the cyst was mansupialized.* **(b)** *Oblique lateral radiograph taken at the same time as Figure 287a.* **(c)** *Two months after operation the cyst has shrunk considerably, taking the tooth upwards and inwards. The mandibular bone has thickened markedly.* **(d)** *Posteroanterior radiograph showing the condition nine months after operation. The tooth has moved upwards and it appears that it may eventually erupt.* **(e)** *An oblique lateral radiograph taken at the same time as Figure 287d showing extensive filling of the cyst cavity with bone.* **(f)** *Three years later the tooth is into occlusion, but is about to be lost due to caries!*

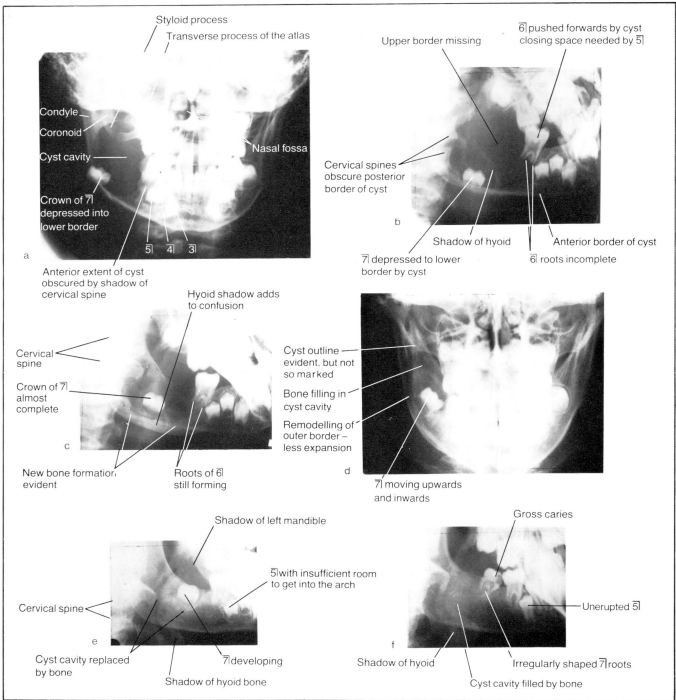

Dentigerous cysts on upper third molars tend to involve the antrum, sometimes almost completely filling the air space (Figure 289). In this case a man aged 19 years had had a discharge of fluid from around the upper molar teeth on the left side. The standard occipitomental radiograph shows a large cyst present filling up the left antral space, the latter being reduced to a very small air space anteriorly, beneath the orbit. There is a vortex of bone covering the upper border of the cyst where it has displaced the antral floor. This enables a differential diagnosis to be made with mucosal retention cyst which does not have a bony covering as it is only related to soft tissue (Figure 303).

Primordial Cyst

Primordial cysts are generally considered to develop from a tooth crypt which fails to develop a calcified structure.

Figure 290 is an oblique lateral radiograph of a woman aged 22 years. There was no history of extrac-

Figure 288. *Oblique lateral and lower occlusal radiograph of a man aged 34 years showing low, horizontal 8̲| with a dentigerous cyst reaching forwards below 76̲| and expanding the bone buccally. The lower cortex has been thinned.*

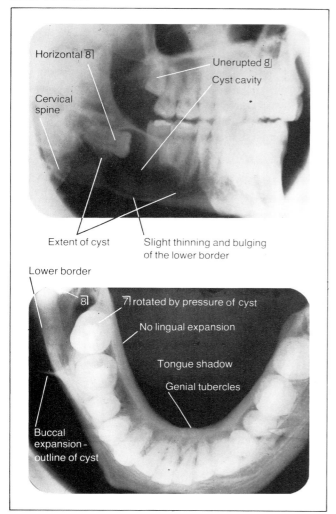

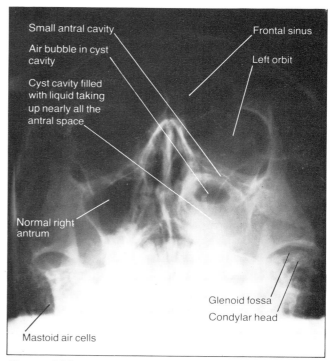

Figure 289. *Occipitomental radiograph of a man aged 19 years showing a large cyst presenting in the left antrum. There is an air bubble inside the cyst cavity; the latter has been open to the mouth for several weeks allowing the cyst lining mucosa to thicken. The small antral cavity can be seen just below the lower margin of the left orbit.*

tion of 8̲| which is absent from the film. Both 76̲| are vital and their laminas are intact. There is a large cystic lesion extending backwards from 6̲| to the sigmoid notch. There is the suggestion of loculation, but this is false, and the impression is created by some of the cortex remaining buccally—the lesion is monolocular.

The diagnosis of primordial cyst was made on these appearances and the histological report. The cyst was

Figure 290. *Oblique lateral radiograph of a woman aged 22 years, showing a cyst-like lesion of the right ramus reaching from the sigmoid notch to 6̲|. Although the radiographic appearance is suggestive of two cavities, this appearance is probably caused by a ridge of cortical bone. 8̲| had never appeared. This is a primordial cyst.*

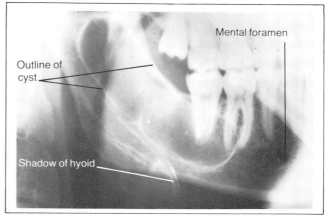

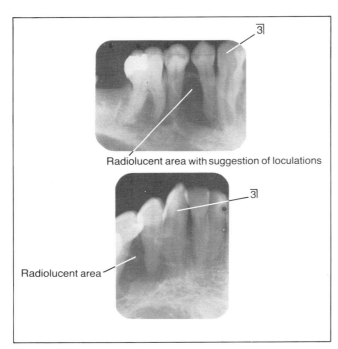

Radiolucent area with suggestion of loculations

Radiolucent area

Figure 291. *Periapical radiographs of a man aged 49 years showing an apparent loculated area of radiolucency with a clearcut margin between 54⌋. Amelo-blastoma should be considered from the radiographic appearance, but the histological report was: 'stratified squamous epithelium with no inflammatory features and not related to 5⌋ or 4⌋'. This is a primordial cyst.*

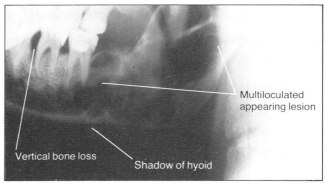

Multiloculated appearing lesion

Vertical bone loss

Shadow of hyoid

Figure 292. *Oblique lateral radiograph of a man aged 36 years showing what appears to be an ameloblastoma of the body and ramus of the left mandible. The multilocular appearance is highly suggestive of this type of lesion, but after two biopsies both pathology reports stated: 'probably primordial cyst—no evidence of neoplasm'.*

operated on, and a year later there had been marked bone replacement in the area.

Another example of primordial cyst is shown in Figure 291. The apparent locular radiolucent area between 54⌋ was investigated and the pathology report stated: 'Attached to the side of the tooth, but not apparently connected with it, is a cyst lined with stratified squamous epithelium and having hyaline bodies and also a microcyst. There are no inflammatory features'. The radiologist's report had suggested the possibility of ameloblastoma.

Even more suggestive of ameloblastoma is Figure 292. The multiloculated appearance of the radiolucent area filling the body of the mandible from ⌊7 region to include the whole ramus is typical of this lesion. The pathology report states: 'not typical of anything—probably a primordial cyst'!

Figure 293. *Oblique lateral and posteroanterior radiographs of a woman aged 63 years showing what appears to be a simple cystic lesion. The lesion 'shelled out' at operation and was found to be a monocystic ameloblastoma—partly solid and partly cystic. The third film shows healing one year later.*

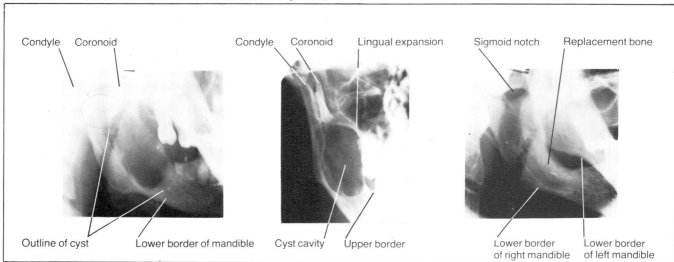

Condyle Coronoid

Outline of cyst   Lower border of mandible

Condyle Coronoid   Lingual expansion

Cyst cavity   Upper border

Sigmoid notch   Replacement bone

Lower border of right mandible   Lower border of left mandible

As a result of this report a thorough exploration and curettage of the bony cavity were made. The second pathology report suggested primordial cyst, and no evidence of neoplasia.

Cystic Neoplasms

Cystic Ameloblastoma

Neoplastic changes within dental or similar cysts are very rare. Cysts forming within ameloblastomas are, however, fairly common.

Figure 292 showed a primordial cyst which exhibited the characteristics of ameloblastoma radiographically. Figure 293 shows a monolocular ameloblastoma which according to the pathology report had a true fluid cyst within the matrix. According to Cawson (1968), once fluid has begun to accumulate within these cysts, the epithelium gets flattened and may become indistinguishable from a simple cyst lining on histological examination. The appearance in Figure 293 is very much that of simple dental cyst, and there is little evidence of the

Figure 294 (a). *Oblique lateral radiograph of a man aged 33 years showing a well-circumscribed radiolucent area related to the apex of $\overline{5}$ and extending backwards to $\overline{7}$ region. The hyoid bone is superimposed and causes some confusion.* **(b)** *Four years later there is a well-defined radiolucent area in $\overline{7}$ region suggesting recurrent or residual cyst.*

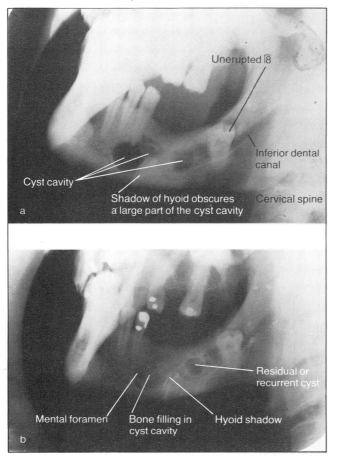

typical multiloculated cystic appearance of ameloblastoma.

Ameloblastoma is considered further in Chapter 8.

Recurrent Cysts

Recurrence of both primordial cyst and cystic ameloblastoma is well documented, and it is worth remembering that if the lining is not entirely removed when enucleating a dental cyst (Figure 294a), it is quite possible for the cystic cavity to heal in part, and then for the cyst to recur (Figure 294b) or continue to develop in the area where the lining has been left.

Non-Odontogenic Cysts

Remnants of epithelium may be left in the tissues during fusion of the embryonic processes giving rise to a number of cysts, most of which appear in the maxilla.

Fissural Cysts

Incisive Canal Cyst

These midline cysts of the maxilla are given a number of names which add to the confusion of diagnosis. They may arise anywhere along the canal from the nasal floor to the palatal mucosa. Radiographically it is seldom possible to determine the exact site of origin, though a true lateral radiograph will often give some indication.

It has been stated that 6 mm probably represents the upper limit of normal diameter, and that an incisive fossa exceeding this size is likely to house a cyst.

Figure 295a to d illustrates examples of incisive canal cysts. They all present as a radiolucency in the midline of the palate, in some cases overlying the roots of the upper incisor teeth. Differential diagnosis with apical cyst of these incisors is not too difficult as the lamina dura will be evident surrounding the apices of vital incisors, and apical cysts of central incisors seldom cross the midline to any extent until they are very large.

The thickness of the cortex of these cysts can vary considerably from very thick to very thin.

In Figure 296 an incisive canal cyst is projected over the apex of $1\rfloor$ due to the positioning technique. The lamina dura can be seen surrounding the apex of this tooth and the tooth was found to be vital. A midline view (Figure 297) clarifies the true position of the cyst.

These cysts are lined with either columnar or stratified squamous epithelium.

Globulomaxillary Cyst (doubtful entity)

This is a rare cyst lined with columnar epithelium which probably arises at the fusion line of embryonic processes, and is best termed a fissural cyst. It presents radiographically as an inverted pear-shaped radiolucency between the roots of the upper lateral incisor and canine (Figure 298), causing wide divergence of these roots. The adjacent teeth will be vital, and in the

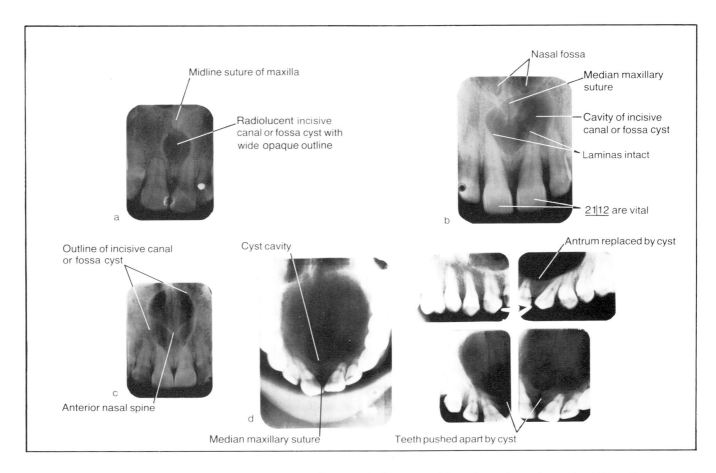

Figure 295 (a). *Periapical radiograph showing small nasopalatine cyst with well-corticated margin. When first noticed radiographically the patient, aged 24 years, had no symptoms. Some time later suppuration occurred.* (b) *Periapical radiograph showing nasopalatine cyst, heart-shaped, at the midline. 1|1 are vital in this man aged 49 years.* (c) *Periapical radiograph showing large nasopalatine cyst with 10 year history of recurrent suppuration in a woman aged 30 years.* (d) *Very large nasopalatine cyst.*

event that they are not, the diagnosis of globulomaxillary cyst must be suspect. Irritation from a secondary root canal, or from a poor periodontal condition could be the cause of a cyst developing in this region.

Figure 296. *Periapical radiograph of a man aged 20 years showing large area of radiolucency over the apex of 1|. The lamina of 1| is intact and this is a nasopalatine cyst in the midline, which appears to be over 1| due to the angle of projection of the x-ray beam.*

Nasolabial Cyst

A nasolabial cyst is generally considered to arise from remnants of epithelium at the area of fusion of the globular, lateral nasal and maxillary processes. It

Figure 297. *Midline radiographic view of the same patient shown in Figure 296. This projection shows the true position of the nasopalatine cyst in the midline.*

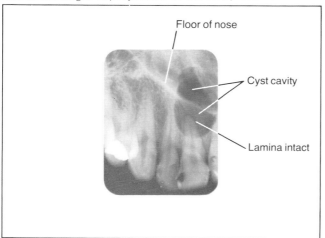

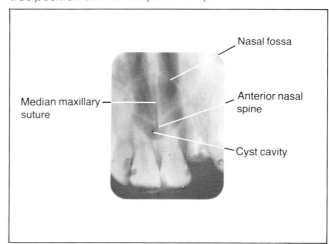

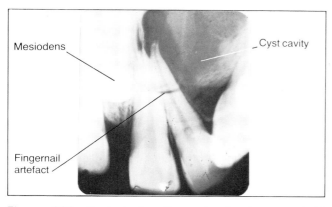

Figure 298. *Periapical radiograph of a boy aged 16 years showing a mesiodens, and so-called globulo-maxillary cyst pushing apices of $\lfloor 23$ apart. A differential diagnosis has to be made with lateral periodontal cyst, and apical cyst on $\lfloor 2$.*

usually presents as a swelling on the mucolabial fold and nostril, and may be lined by either columnar or stratified squamous epithelium.

It can be shown best radiographically by injecting lipiodol (a radio-opaque oil) into the cyst cavity having first removed some of the contents (Figure 299a and b). Without the lipiodol the cyst would not show up well as it does not involve bone.

Median Mandibular Cyst

Inclusion cysts developing in the suture line between the two halves of the mandible are very rare indeed and tend to enlarge symmetrically from the midline. They can occur low down near the lower border of the mandible

Figure 299 (a). *Lateral skull radiograph showing naso-labial cyst cavity injected with lipiodol to show the full extent of the lesion.* **(b)** *Oblique upper occlusal radiograph showing the same cyst cavity outlined by lipiodol.*

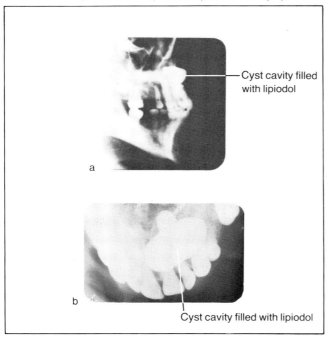

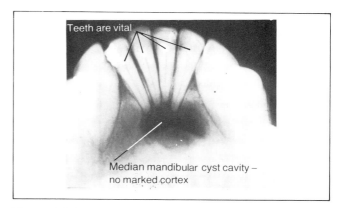

Figure 300. *Lower oblique anterior occlusal radiograph of a man aged 39 years demonstrating a median cyst of the mandible. All anterior teeth were found to be vital when tested by two operators. The patient attended for treatment as a result of infection of the cyst.*

in which case they are unlikely to be mistaken for cysts arising from teeth.

In Figure 300 the cyst has developed higher up in the mandible and reached the apices of $\overline{21|12}$. The 39-year-old man attended with discomfort in this region and the teeth were tested for vitality as the lesion was assumed to be an apical periodontal cyst. Several tests were made, all of which proved positive and, because the surgeon was still suspicious, pits were drilled in the back of the teeth to make quite certain that all the teeth were vital. They were. This is a median mandibular cyst.

Non-epithelialized Bone Cyst

Figure 301 depicts a solitary bone cyst in the mandible of a girl aged 12 years. This was a chance radiographical finding, and following surgery there was infilling of the cavity by bone. The diagnosis of non-epithelialized bone cyst was made from the pathology report.

Figure 301. *Periapical radiographs of a girl aged 12 years showing non-epithelialized bone cyst. This was a chance radiological finding, and the diagnosis was made after the operation, following receipt of the pathology report.*

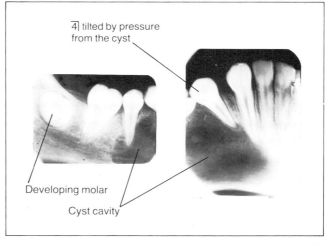

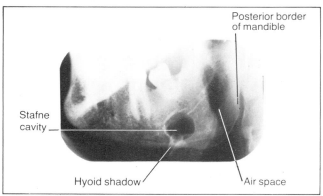

Figure 302. *Oblique lateral radiograph of left mandible showing Stafne cavity.*

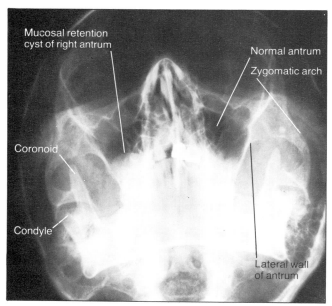

Figure 303. *Standard occipitomental view of a woman aged 56 years showing a mucosal retention cyst in the lower part of the right antrum. There is no bone covering the 'dome' of the cyst, and this helps in the differential diagnosis with a dental cyst pushing the antrum aside.*

Stafne Cavity or Latent Bone Cyst

Latent bone cysts have already been discussed in Chapter 2. They are generally accepted as depressions in the mandible with salivary or connective tissue contents, and may well resemble a cyst radiographically (Figure 302).

Antral Mucosal Retention Cyst

These soft tissue retention cysts frequently present as a chance finding on radiographs and are particularly well shown on the standard occipitomental projection (Figure 303). They are symptomless in most cases and are left to subside without intervention. It is necessary to make a differential diagnosis with periodontal or dentigerous cyst displacing the antrum (Figures 289 and 304). In the original radiograph a bony covering (the antral floor) can be seen overlying the convexity of the

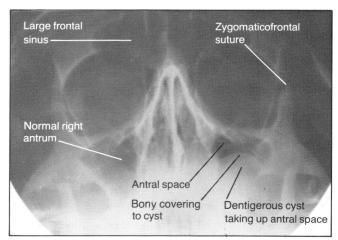

Figure 304. *Occipitomental radiographic view illustrating dentigerous cyst (related to $\lfloor 8$) occupying most of the left antral space. The bony antral floor overlying the cyst can be seen on the original radiograph and serves to distinguish this type of cyst from mucosal retention cyst.*

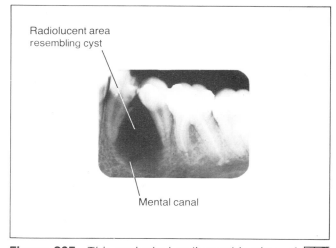

Figure 305. *This periapical radiographic view of $\lceil 4\text{-}7$ region depicts a large radiolucent area pushing aside the apices of $\lceil 45$. This looks very much like a cyst. $\lceil 45$ were vital and the pathology report stated: 'dental granuloma'!*

upper border of the cyst in Figure 304. In the mucosal cyst there is no bony covering evident on the radiograph as this is a soft tissue cyst of the lining mucosa of the antrum.

Problems in Diagnosis of Cysts

It is by no means always possible to make a certain diagnosis of cyst from the radiographic evidence alone, and histological examination is normally required. Figure 305 suggests a cyst between $\lceil 45$ in a girl aged 17 years, and the surgeon made this provisional diagnosis, although $\lceil 45$ appeared to be vital. The pathology report stated that this was a dental granuloma!

References

Cawson, R. A., *Essentials of Dental Surgery and Pathology*, Churchill, London, 1968.

8. Neoplasms and Tumour-like Lesions of the Jaws

Dental practitioners are unlikely to see many malignant neoplasms during their lifetime, but it is important that they should be able to recognize the radiographic signs of malignancy and refer their patients appropriately as soon as possible.

Radiographs of any suspected tumour should include the whole extent of the lesion and the margin of the surrounding tissues. In many cases this will mean extra-oral radiographs taken at oblique angles such as oblique laterals, occipitofrontals and occipitomentals. Panoramic radiographs are of great help in showing the full extent of lesions of the mandible, but the use of intensifying screens and the rotational movement of the tubehead and film result in some loss of definition on the radiograph as a result of blurring.

Where possible, intra-oral views using periapical and occlusal film should be taken, as the margins of lesions, which are so significant, can be seen in better detail.

Benign neoplasms generally depict a sharp image margin in bone. They tend to enlarge slowly, pushing against the bone to cause expansion, and may produce radiolucent, opaque or mixed density images on radiographs.

Malignant neoplasms present an invasive picture, infiltrating the surrounding tissues. Radiographically the bony margin is poorly defined, and sometimes missing altogether where the cortex has been invaded and destroyed.

Metastases from the bronchus, breast, kidney and prostate may present in the jaws and may be lytic or sclerotic in appearance.

Many neoplasms present an indeterminate radiographic appearance and, in the end, a diagnosis may be resolved only by a pathology report following biopsy or excision. It is the radiologist's job to recognize neoplasia as such. He may, or may not, be able to indicate the likely histological structure from the radiographic appearance alone. Table 3 gives a suitable classification when considering the radiographic appearance of tumours of the jaws.

Table 3. Classification of neoplasms and tumour-like lesions.

Benign Epithelial Neoplasms	*Benign Mesothelial Neoplasms*
Odontogenic	Odontogenic
Enameloma	Fibroma
Ameloblastoma	Cementoma
Recurrent ameloblastoma	Dentinoma
Melanotic ameloblastoma	Non-Odontogenic
Non-Odontogenic	Fibroma —peripheral and central
Adenoma and pleomorphic adenoma	Ossifying fibroma, fibro-esteoma
	Osteoma —Tori, exosteal, endosteal
Benign Mixed Neoplasms	Chondroma and chondro-osteoma
Mineralized	Osteoclastoma —peripheral and central
Dilated and invaginated odontome	Haemangioma —capillary and
Geminated odontome	cavernous
Complex odontome	Eosinophilic granuloma
Compound odontome	Neurofibroma
Part Mineralized	
Teratoma	*Malignant Mesothelial Neoplasms*
Non-Mineralized	Osteogenic
Fibro-ameloblastoma	Fibrosarcoma
	Chondrosarcoma
Malignant Epithelial Neoplasms	Osteosarcoma
Odontogenic	Non-osteogenic
Epithelioma from dental remnants —rare	Malignant neurofibroma
Non-odontogenic	Myosarcoma
Carcinoma	Liposarcoma
Metastases	Myeloma
Melanoma	Lymphosarcoma
Adenocarcinoma	

Benign Epithelial Neoplasms

Odontogenic Neoplasms

Enameloma

This overgrowth of enamel, generally found near the bifurcation of molar roots as a small enamel 'pearl', has already been described in the article on developmental abnormalities (Chapter 2).

Ameloblastoma

The majority of these tumours arise in the mandible near the angle. They are usually slow-growing, locally invasive, and tend to recur. Radiographically they may be multi-loculated in appearance (Figure 306a), the loculations being separated by bony trabeculations of different thicknesses, though it is not unknown for these tumours to appear to be unilocular. In the latter case the margin is generally lobulated.

Figure 306b illustrates the erosion of related roots and lamina dura of $\overline{56}$ and the multi-cystic appearance of this lesion. Figure 306c shows the marked lingual expansion resulting from this tumour in a woman aged 31 years. In all three radiographic views the periphery of the bony outline appears to be intact, and there is no sign of any periosteal reaction.

Downgrowth of the tumour to involve the lower border of the mandible poses a problem for the surgeon, as incomplete removal of the tumour will result in continued growth of the remnants.

Figure 307a is an oblique lateral radiograph of a man aged 31 years showing an apparent single-cystic type ameloblastoma. On careful examination of the original radiograph smaller circular areas of deeper radiolucency can be seen within the larger radiolucency. The cortex of the lower border has been thinned and there is the suggestion of the resorption of the roots of $\overline{6}$. The tumour was enucleated. Fifteen months later (Figure 207b), although there has been some bone regeneration distally at the lower border of the lesion, there is a recurrence. Small circular 'daughter' cysts can be seen with fragments of radiopaque dressing lying nearby. Two years later still the tumour has greatly increased in size (Figure 307c), has a cystic appearance, and has again reached the lower border. There is marked resorption of the distal root of $\overline{6}$ and this tooth has distal caries. The radiographic appearance of the tumour has changed considerably since Figure 307a.

Figure 308 shows a recurrent ameloblastoma of the

Figure 306 (a). *Oblique lateral view of a multicystic ameloblastoma in a woman aged 31 years, showing displacement upwards of $\overline{56}$. The lesion extends upwards to the coronoid process and condyle, and down to involve the lower border of the mandible. The varying sized loculations are well outlined. (b) Intra-oral periapical radiographic views of the same patient showing resorption of the roots of $\overline{56}$ and displacement of these teeth upwards. There is no suggestion of a cortex in the radiolucent area beneath $\overline{56}$, but there is the suggestion of both cortex and trabeculations further back in the third molar region. (c) Lower occlusal view showing marked lingual expansion with 'lobular' bony outline to the lesion and irregular trabeculation. There is no sign of periosteal reaction in any of the views.*

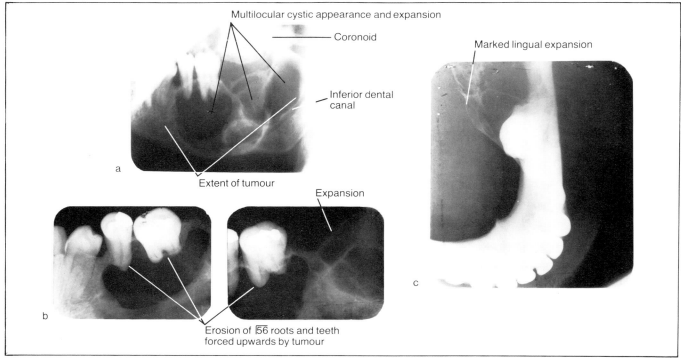

mandible in a man aged 65 years. He had had a number of unsuccessful operations for removal of the tumour over a period of 20 years. The typical 'daughter' cysts of recurrent ameloblastoma are evident and must be distinguished from myeloma deposits. Ameloblastomas are said not to metastasize (though metastases have been found), whereas myeloma deposits will nearly always be found in a number of bones.

Figure 307 (a). *Oblique lateral view of an ameloblastoma in a man aged 31 years. The appearance is monolocular, though darker areas can be seen within the radiolucency on the original radiograph, suggesting possible loculations. The margins are circumscribed and well outlined, reaching down to the lower border.* **(b)** *After operation there is recurrence 15 months later, or more likely continuance, of the lesion. A number of 'daughter' cysts are evident below $\overline{6|}$. Bone regeneration has taken place both at the lower border and forwards to the mesial root of $\overline{7|}$. The opaque spots are fragments of dressing left after the operation.* **(c)** *Resorption of distal root of $\overline{6|}$ is evident, and there is marked extension of the lesion two years later. The lower border is again involved.*

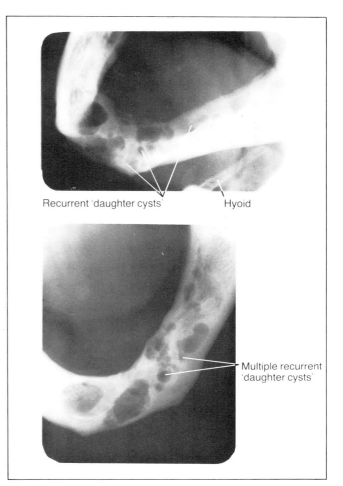

Recurrent 'daughter cysts'   Hyoid

Multiple recurrent 'daughter cysts'

Figure 308. *Oblique lateral and occlusal radiographs of the left mandible of a man aged 65 years. He had a history of ameloblastoma over a period of 20 years with a number of resections, each followed by recurrence. The typical multiple 'daughter' cysts can be seen extending from $\overline{3|}$ to $\overline{|7}$ region. Differential diagnosis has to be made with multiple myeloma.*

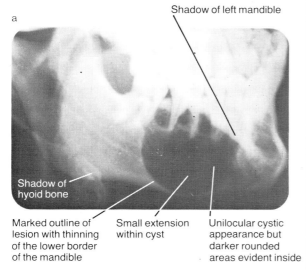

a

Shadow of left mandible

Shadow of hyoid bone

Marked outline of lesion with thinning of the lower border of the mandible

Small extension within cyst

Unilocular cystic appearance but darker rounded areas evident inside

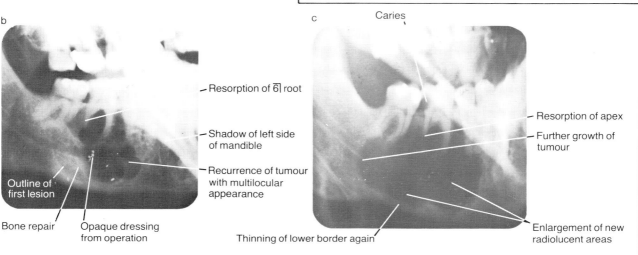

b

Outline of first lesion

Bone repair   Opaque dressing from operation

Resorption of $\overline{6|}$ root

Shadow of left side of mandible

Recurrence of tumour with multilocular appearance

c   Caries

Resorption of apex

Further growth of tumour

Thinning of lower border again

Enlargement of new radiolucent areas

115

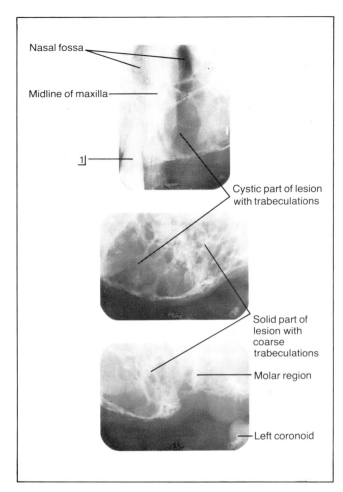

Figure 309. *Intra-oral radiographs of a man aged 38 years, showing ameloblastoma of the 'solid' type extending from the midline to the molar region. The lesion does not appear to have crossed the midline at this stage though it has reached it. There is the suggestion of a cystic portion in the incisor region, the appearance changing to a smaller honeycombed pattern further back in the maxilla. A cortex is still evident outside the lesion, though it is rather irregular in outline.*

Some ameloblastomas are 'solid' in appearance and Figure 309 represents such a case. The patient, a man aged 38 years, had a lesion extending from the midline to the left molar region of the maxilla. The small variable-sized radiolucencies surrounded by a cortex present a honeycombed appearance less definite than that generally outlining benign tumours or cysts. Often these 'solid' ameloblastomas contain cystic portions as well.

Melanotic Ameloblastoma

Figure 310 is an intra-oral radiograph of BA|AB region of a girl aged six months showing this intra-osseous destructive radiolucent lesion. The bone outline is evident though not marked. These tumours are said to

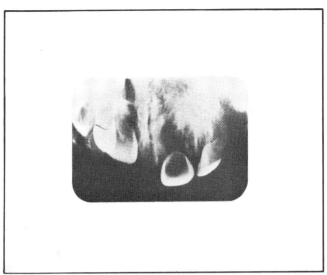

Figure 310. *Intra-oral radiograph of BA|AB region, showing apparent extrusion of developing |AB and related bone destruction. The round firm lesion was excised and contained black patches of melanin on section. There was no evidence of recurrence 15 years later. The pathological report was 'melanotic ameloblastoma' in this six-month-old girl.*

arise before the child reaches six months of age, and are sometimes termed retinal anlage or melanotic progonoma. There was no evidence of any recurrence when the patient had reached 16 years of age.

Non-Odontogenic Neoplasms

Adenoma and Pleomorphic Adenoma

Tumours containing salivary gland tissue are occasionally found in the jaws, most often in the parotid gland itself. Figure 311a shows the duct system of a normal right submandibular gland outlined with lipiodol—an oil-based contrast medium obtained from Poppy seeds.

Figure 311b shows the duct system of a 62-year-old man with a history of a swelling of the right submandibular gland of five years duration. There is forward enlargement of the gland and loss of duct structure between the main ducts, which have been forced apart by the tumour. The shadow of the hyoid bone can be seen superimposed on the centre of the gland. The pathology report stated: 'Pleomorphic adenoma'. It should be remembered that these tumours can become malignant.

Benign Mesothelial Neoplasms

Odontogenic Neoplasms

Odontogenic Fibroma and Myxoma

These rare tumours arise from the tooth follicle, dental papilla or periodontal membrane. They are generally

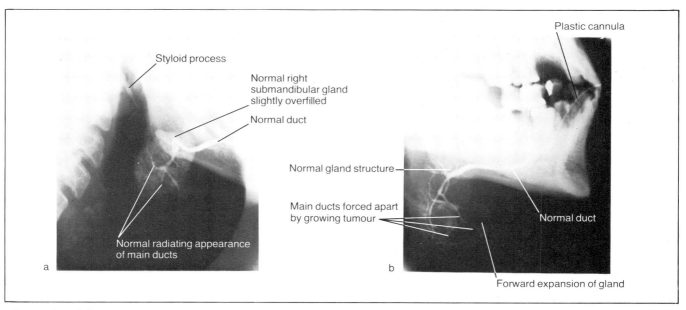

Figure 311 (a). *Normal right submandibular gland sialogram using lipiodol as the contrast medium. The gland alveoli are slightly overfilled.* **(b)** *Right submandibular sialogram of a patient aged 62 years with a history of swelling in this region of five years duration. There is expansion within the gland pushing the large ducts apart, and enclosing areas of radiolucency with no duct structure. The pathology report stated 'Pleomorphic adenoma'.*

radiolucent, close to a tooth, and encapsulated (Figure 312). In this case, a man aged 29 years, the cortex of the lower border of the mandible is thinned on the inner aspect, the ⌐6 roots are short and eroded. Note the marked cystic appearance and cortical outline to the lesion.

Odontogenic myxoma is thought likely, in some instances, to be a mucoid degeneration of an odontogenic fibroma.

Cementoma

True cementoma has to be differentiated from periapical osteofibrosis, and hypercementosis arising from

Figure 312. *Part of a Panelipse radiograph of a man aged 29 years with an odontogenic fibroma. The radiolucent area beneath ⌐6 reaches the lower border and appears cyst-like, but the outline cortex is not quite as smooth as that of a cyst. ⌐6 roots appear short, probably due to resorption. The third molars are unable to erupt into the arch due to overcrowding.*

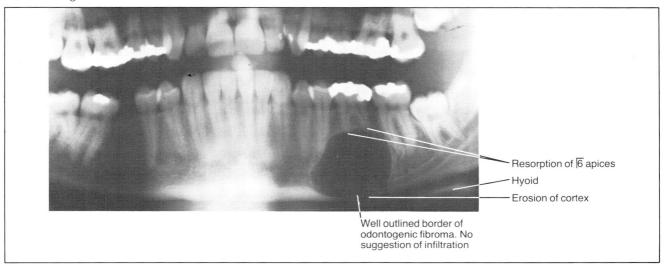

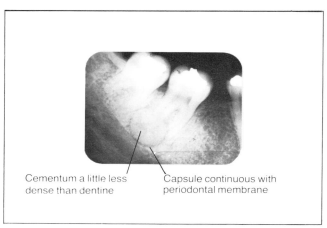

Cementum a little less dense than dentine

Capsule continuous with periodontal membrane

Figure 313. *Periapical radiograph of a man aged 25 years showing a cementoma at the distal apex of* 7⌐. *The surrounding capsule is continuous with the periodontal membrane, and the tumour is slightly less opaque than the dentine.*

irritation or infection. Cementoma is a rare tumour appearing as a bulbous growth of cementum on the apex during the formation of a tooth. Figure 313 demonstrates cementoma at the distal apex of 7⌐ in a man aged 25 years. The lesion is well-rounded and is surrounded by a radiolucent fibrous capsule continuous with the periodontal membrane shadow of this tooth.

Dentinoma

This is a very rare tumour composed of dentine, sometimes also containing connective tissue. Radiologically it resembles a simple odontome.

Non-Odontogenic Neoplasms

Fibroma

Peripheral fibroma, also sometimes termed 'epulis' is a superficial common growth in the mouth. It is seldom noticed radiologically unless there has been some ossification. Figure 314a, b, c and d shows four examples of peripheral fibromas with ossification. The outline of the soft tissue mass can be seen on the original radiograph in Figure 314d. It is interesting to note that in each case there has been local loss of supporting bone, but no union of the new bone with the maxilla or mandible.

Central fibromas are rare, mainly appearing in the mandible. The example seen in Figure 315, however, is in the left maxilla, in a boy aged 12 years. There has been expansion of the maxilla, but the tumour has not

Figure 314 (a). *Peripheral fibroma with ossification in* 8⌐ *region. The soft tissue of the lesion is also visible on this oblique lateral radiograph.* **(b)** *Peripheral fibroma with ossification in* ⌐6 *region.* **(c)** *Peripheral fibroma with ossification evident on a true occlusal radiograph of a patient aged 30 years.* **(d)** *Peripheral fibroma with ossification evident on intra-oral radiograph of a man aged 26 years.*

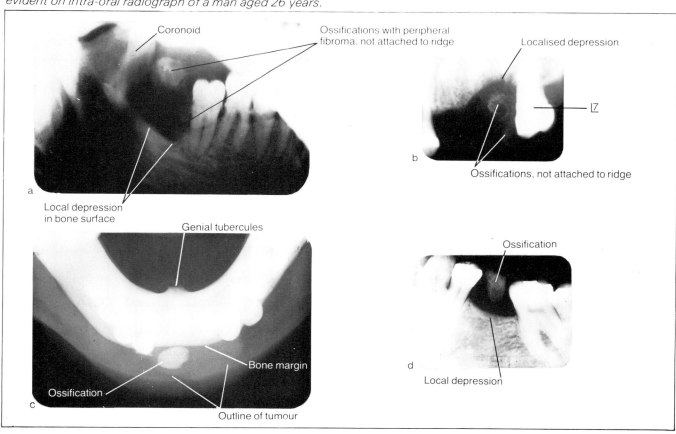

Coronoid

Ossifications with peripheral fibroma, not attached to ridge

Localised depression

⌐7

Ossifications, not attached to ridge

Local depression in bone surface

Genial tubercules

Ossification

Bone margin

Local depression

Ossification

Outline of tumour

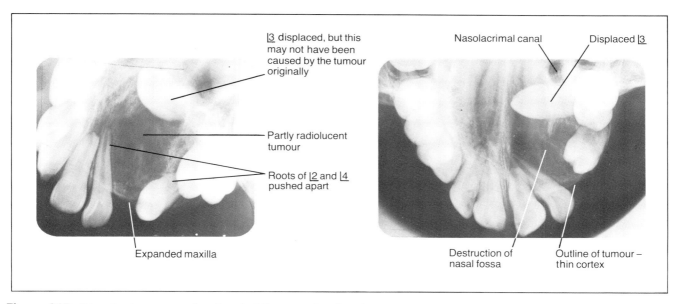

Nasolacrimal canal

Displaced |3

|3 displaced, but this may not have been caused by the tumour originally

Partly radiolucent tumour

Roots of |2 and |4 pushed apart

Expanded maxilla

Destruction of nasal fossa

Outline of tumour – thin cortex

Figure 315. *Standard upper occlusal and oblique occlusal radiographs of a boy aged 12 years with a central fibroma. There is swelling of |1-5 region and the related teeth have been pushed well apart, particularly the roots. There is the suggestion of loculation or lobulation, and some fine trabeculation is still evident. |3 is markedly displaced.*

crossed the midline. There is marked displacement of the related teeth with little sign of a well corticated border of the rather radiolucent lesion. Some destruction of the left nasal fossa is also evident.

Ossifying Fibroma or Fibro-osteoma

These tumours are often regarded nowadays as a form of fibrous dysplasia, though the matter is not settled for certain.

Figures 316 and 317 show two cases of ossifying fibroma of the mandible. In Figure 316 there has been marked buccal expansion of the mandible, the inferior dental canal has been depressed well down to the lower border, the ossification is granular in appearance, and a narrow white line outlines the tumour.

Figure 317 shows no expansion of the mandible, but depicts a wide capsule surrounding the irregularly outlined lesion in this woman aged 53 years.

A large ossifying fibroma of the maxilla in a woman

Figure 316. *Oblique lateral and occlusal radiographs of a man aged 48 years with ossifying fibroma of the left mandible. The mandibular canal has been pushed downwards, and a white line can be seen surrounding the granular appearing bone. At first sight there appears to be a radiolucent capsule on the oblique lateral view, but this is probably the outline of the depressed mandibular canal. The lesion was very slow growing, and was trimmed to a convenient size and shape.*

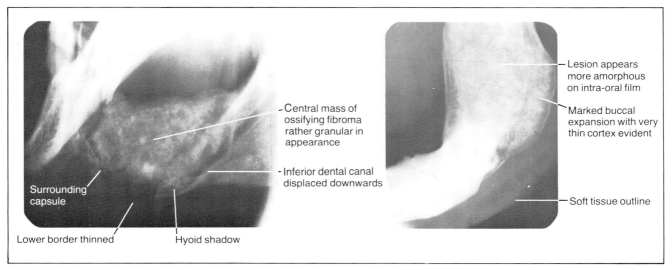

Central mass of ossifying fibroma rather granular in appearance

Inferior dental canal displaced downwards

Surrounding capsule

Lower border thinned

Hyoid shadow

Lesion appears more amorphous on intra-oral film

Marked buccal expansion with very thin cortex evident

Soft tissue outline

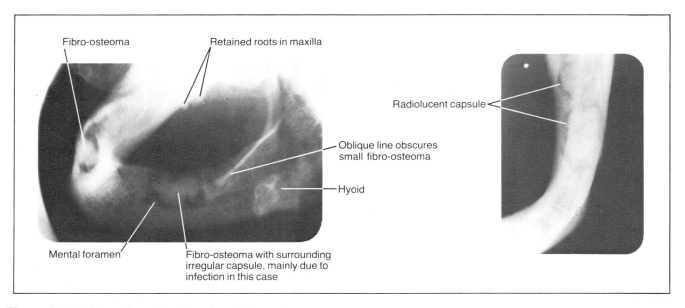

Fibro-osteoma

Retained roots in maxilla

Radiolucent capsule

Oblique line obscures small fibro-osteoma

Hyoid

Mental foramen

Fibro-osteoma with surrounding irregular capsule, mainly due to infection in this case

Figure 317. *Oblique lateral and occlusal views of a woman aged 53 years with an ossifying fibroma, or fibro-osteoma. The irregularly outlined lesion exhibits much the same density as cortical bone and is surrounded by a radiolucent capsule. The area had become infected. A second lesion can be seen on the occlusal radiograph behind the large one, and a third is evident on the oblique lateral view near the midline.*

aged 36 years is shown in Figure 318. It occupies almost the entire antral space and has expanded the lateral wall.

Osteoma

Torus palatinus and torus mandibularis are sometimes described as osteomas, and sclerosing osteitis is sometimes misdiagnosed as osteoma. Osteomas are termed exosseous when they arise from the periosteum (Figure 319), and endosseous when they arise from the endo-

steum. Many of the dense bone islands, which are described in Chapter 2, are a form of endosteal osteoma.

Osteomas can present as 'ivory' or 'compact' osteomas (Figure 319) or 'cancellous' osteomas (Figure 320).

Figure 319. *Occlusal radiographic views of ivory osteomas on the buccal and lingual surfaces of the mandible respectively. The marked density of the lesions is apparent, and both are pedunculated.*

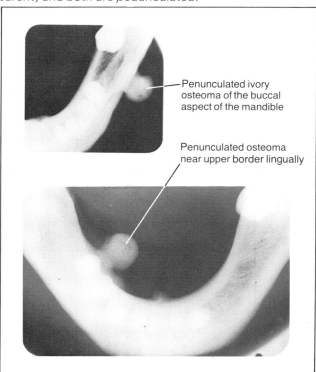

Penunculated ivory osteoma of the buccal aspect of the mandible

Penunculated osteoma near upper border lingually

Figure 318. *Occipitomental view of a woman aged 36 years with an ossifying fibroma of the right maxilla, taking up most of the antral space, and expanding the lateral antral wall.*

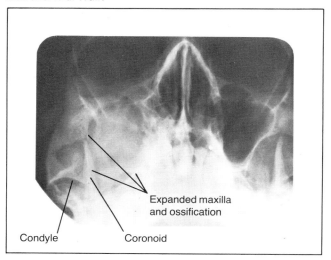

Expanded maxilla and ossification

Condyle   Coronoid

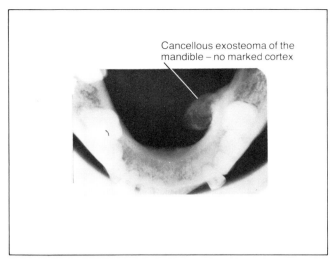

Figure 320. *Occlusal view of a cancellous osteoma of the mandible of a woman aged 40 years. The trabecular pattern is evident and the cortex is unpronounced.*

Multiple osteomas are sometimes seen, and Figure 321 demonstrates a multiple osteoma of the maxilla in a man aged 67 years. These lesions can interfere with the stability of dentures, and in some instances their removal is indicated.

Chondroma and Chondro-osteoma

Chondroma is a tumour of cartilage which is very rare in the jaws, but when present may become malignant. Radiographic appearances are inconsistent, though the lesions are generally radiolucent and cyst-like, with or without expansion. If there is partial ossification within the tumour there is difficulty in the differential diagnosis with chondro-osteoma.

Figure 322 is part of a posteroanterior radiograph of a woman with a chondro-osteoma of the lateral surface of the base of the right condyle, a common site for this uncommon lesion.

Figure 321. *Upper standard occlusal view of a man aged 67 years illustrating multiple cancellous osteomas of the maxilla.*

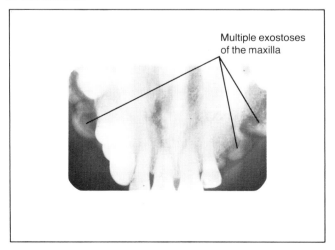

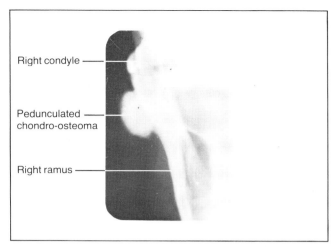

Figure 322. *Part of a posteroanterior view of an opaque chondro-osteoma at the base of the right condyle of a woman. This was removed surgically but did not cure the clicking joint that had originally brought the patient for treatment!*

Osteoclastoma

Peripheral benign giant cell reparative granuloma, giant cell epulis, and myeloid epulis all signify the same lesion.

Generally there are no radiographic changes evident on the bone adjacent to this soft tissue mass, though occasionally they produce saucer-shaped depressions, of variable depth, in the bone (Figure 323) on radiographic

Figure 323. *Intra-oral periapical views of ⌊67 region of a woman aged 35 years, showing a depression in the alveolus caused by a peripheral giant cell granuloma. The lesion does not involve the antrum; the apparent superimposition is caused by the angle of projection of the x-rays.*

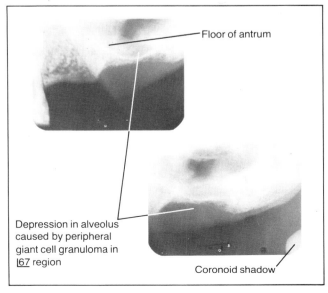

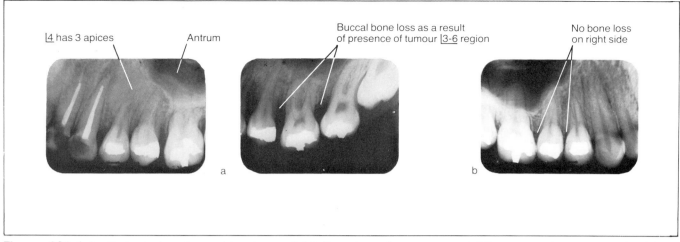

Figure 324 (a). *Periapical radiographic views of ⌊3-7 region of a man aged 20 years, who presented with a pedunculated swelling in ⌊3-6 region of three months duration. There is bone change at the apices of root treated ⌊23, and at the apex of ⌊4, which appears to have three roots. In addition there is considerable alveolar bone loss in ⌊3-7 region which is related to the giant cell reparative granuloma in this area.* **(b)** *Periapical radiograph 6-3⌋ region of the same patient showing normal alveolar bone of the opposite side, and a 3-rooted 4⌋.*

projections. On occasions the alveolar crest may be lost as is seen in Figure 324a in ⌊3-6 region, where some buccal crest bone has been lost. Compare this with the opposite side of the mouth (Figure 324b) in this man aged 20 years.

It is said (Worth 1963) that giant cell epulis is more likely to produce bone loss than the fibroid variety.

Central benign giant cell reparative granuloma tends to occur in the younger patient, often before 20 years of age, and sometimes after a history of previous trauma. Some present with a well defined area of bone destruction radiographically (Figure 325a and b), apparently unilocular, with no sign of trabeculations or cortex. A small buccal expansion with a very thin cortex was evident on the occlusal radiograph of this man aged 24 years (not shown), and this helps in making the diagnosis. Differential diagnosis has to be made with non-epithelialized bone cyst, where there is unlikely to be any expansion of the cortex.

A peripheral film taken one year later (Figure 325c) shows healing, with new bone formation, following removal of the 'tumour'. The roots of 54⌋ have remained separated.

Other giant cell reparative granulomas have less well-defined margins (Figure 326) with the bony outline missing in some places, and show numerous fine or coarse irregular ridges on the surface. The bony expanded covering tends to be undulating rather than smooth, and this helps in the differential diagnosis with cyst. There is often resorption of the roots of related teeth. In this particular case, a girl aged nine years, there is marked displacement of ⌊134, and no sign of ⌊2.

Figure 325 (a). *Periapical view of 654⌋ region of a woman aged 24 years with a central giant cell reparative granuloma between 54⌋ roots. The lamina on these teeth adjacent to the lesion has been thinned and the roots of the teeth have been forced apart. There is little evidence of trabeculation.* **(b)** *Occlusal view of the same patient showing the radiolucent lesion reaching the lateral incisor lingually, and buccal expansion with thin cortex between 54⌋.* **(c)** *Bone regeneration following surgical removal of the lesion and reformation of the lamina round 54⌋, in the same patient as (a) and (b).*

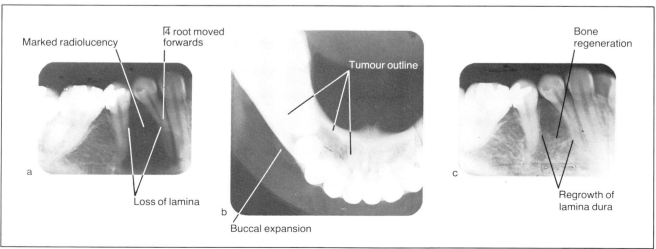

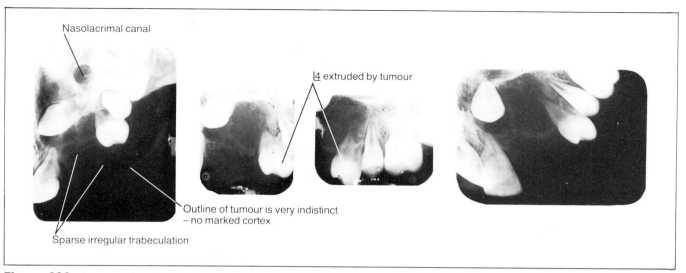

Figure 326. *Intra-oral radiographs of a girl aged nine years with a central giant cell reparative granuloma of the maxilla. There is marked expansion of the maxilla and displacement of the related teeth. Some trabeculations can be seen suggesting loculations, but the outline of the lesion is somewhat indistinct. There is no obvious resorption of the related tooth roots.*

The giant cell tumour of hyperparathyroidism is indistinguishable from the central giant cell reparative granuloma, so the lamina dura surrounding the teeth in the rest of the jaws should be checked carefully whenever such lesions are discovered.

Haemangioma

This rare neoplasm presents in two forms: capillary or cavernous. Radiographic appearances are variable and the condition may not show at all when superficial.

Figure 327 illustrates a capillary haemangioma of the maxilla in a man aged 25 years. There is some destruction of the bone crest between ⌊12, between the apices ⌊23 and at the apex of ⌊3. There is slight

resorption of the lamina at the mesial aspect of ⌊3 apex. However, there is little else radiographically to lead to the diagnosis of capillary haemangioma.

Cavernous haemangioma may present as seen in Figure 328. The soft tissue spaces are very variable in size though generally spherical in outline. The tra-

Figure 328. *Oblique lateral and intra-oral radiographic views of a man aged 53 years with a cavernous haemangioma of the chin and left side of the face, reaching to the angle of the mandible. The lesion had been present for a period of 15 years. There was a hard lobulated swelling in the buccal sulcus and the biopsy report was 'Cavernous haemangioma'. The soft tissue spaces evident on the radiograph are very variable in size and the lamina dura of the tooth sockets is largely missing.*

Figure 327. *Periapical view of ⌊23 region in a man aged 25 years with a capillary haemangioma of ⌊1-3 region. There is some destruction of the bone crest between ⌊12, between ⌊23 apices, and at ⌊3 apex with slight erosion on the mesial aspect. There are no other radiographic changes evident on this region.*

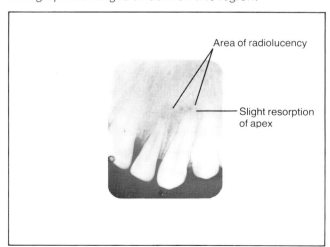

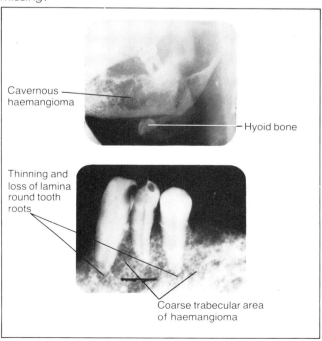

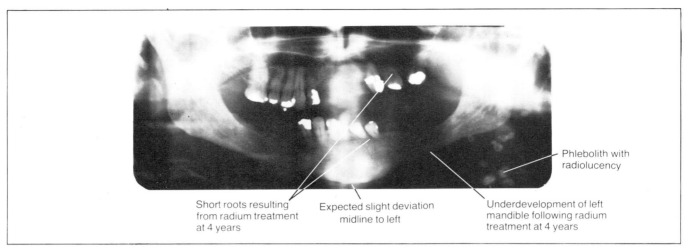

Phlebolith with radiolucency

Short roots resulting from radium treatment at 4 years

Expected slight deviation midline to left

Underdevelopment of left mandible following radium treatment at 4 years

Figure 329. *Panelipse radiograph of a woman aged 40 years with a cavernous haemangioma of the left side of the face and neck containing phleboliths. These calcifications are frequently found in this condition and present as opacities with a small eccentric radiolucency within. Undergrowth of the left side of the mandible and underdevelopment of the teeth on the same side have followed as a result of radium treatment to the lesion when the patient was four years of age. The midline of the mandible has swung slightly to the patient's left as a result of this undergrowth.*

ditional appearance of the horizontal trabeculations of a normal mandible is absent, as is the lamina dura of the teeth related to the lesion. The patient concerned, a man aged 53 years, had involvement of the chin and left side of the face extending to the angle of the mandible. In addition there was hard lobulated swelling of the left buccal sulcus.

Phleboliths in a cavernous haemangioma involving the left intra-oral tissue and the neck of a woman aged 40 years are shown in Figure 329. The patient had had radium treatment for the lesion when aged four years. Multiple smallish opaque round and oval bodies with an eccentric radiolucent dot are well depicted and indicate the condition. A differential diagnosis has to be made

with the concretions of salivary calculi, but this should not prove difficult when multiple opacities are evident. In addition, salivary calculi are often laminated.

Haemangioma are congenital in many cases and they pose a problem in surgery because of the considerable bleeding that occurs.

Eosinophilic Granuloma

Eosinophilic granuloma is thought to be an inflammatory reaction of the reticulo-endothelial tissues of bone. It occurs mainly in the mandible of older children and young adults, though the lesions may be multiple, as is seen in Hand-Schüller-Christian disease. The radio-

Figure 330. *Posteroanterior and oblique lateral views of a man aged 31 years. He had had recurrent swelling and pain in the region of the left ramus. A well-marked circular radiolucency can be seen behind the inferior dental canal towards the back of the left ramus. On the posteroanterior view the outline of the lesion appears more irregular and the cortex buccally is eroded. The biopsy reported 'Histiocytes amongst which are many eosinophyls'. This is an example of eosinophylic granuloma.*

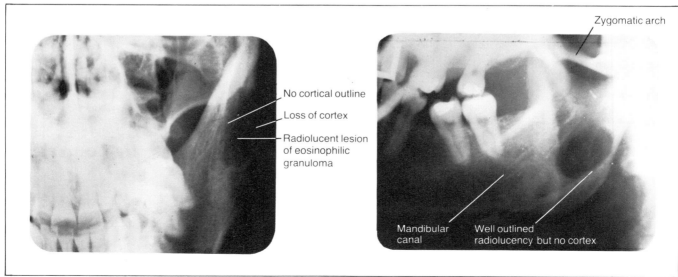

No cortical outline

Loss of cortex

Radiolucent lesion of eosinophilic granuloma

Zygomatic arch

Mandibular canal

Well outlined radiolucency but no cortex

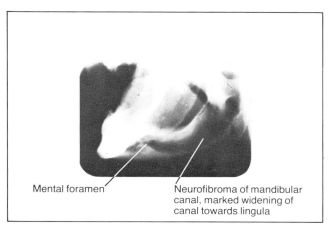

Mental foramen | Neurofibroma of mandibular canal, marked widening of canal towards lingula

Figure 331. *Oblique lateral radiographic view of the left mandible of a woman aged 60 years with a marked widening of the mandibular canal from the mental foramen back to the lingula. She had paraesthesia of the lip but no other signs of this neurofibroma.*

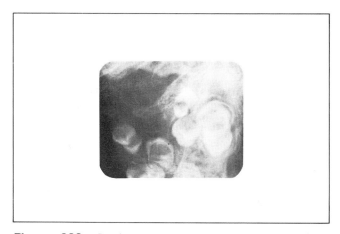

Figure 332. *Radiograph of part of a benign cystic teratoma in a ruptured ovary of a girl aged 10 years. There were many cysts present — also hair follicles, nerve tissue, cartilage and fat, in addition to many developing teeth.*

graphic appearance of eosinophilic granuloma shows well demarcated radiolucent lesions with destruction of the adjacent cortex (Figure 330). This 31-year-old man had a history of recurrent swelling and pain in the left ramus. A section from the lesion showed fibrous tissue with histiocytes and related eosinophils, and lymphocytes.

Neurofibroma

These tumours arise from the fibrous tissue sheath of nerves, and may appear in multiple form (neurofibromatosis). When related to the jaws they may arise subperiosteally, centrally, or within the inferior dental canal. When in the canal they appear as a fusiform or round radiolucency expanding the canal, sometimes to erode the cortex. Figure 331 illustrates a neurofibroma of the inferior dental canal of a woman aged 60 who had paraesthesia of the lip. There were no other clinical symptoms or signs of the tumour.

Benign Mixed Neoplasms

Mineralized Neoplasms

The Odontomes

Odontomes have already been discussed in Chapter 2. These tumours include dilated and invaginated odontomes, geminated odontomes, complex odontomes, and compound odontomes.

Mixture of Mineralized and Non-Mineralized Neoplasms

Teratoma

This neoplasm is mentioned here due to the occasional presence of normal-looking and rudimentary teeth in teratoma of the ovary. The benign teratoma may con-

tain epithelium, hair and teeth, and the ovary and testes are common sites: however, teratomas of the testes are more predisposed to malignancy than those of the ovary. Figure 332 illustrates part of a benign cystic teratoma of the ruptured ovary of a girl aged 10 years. The ovary contained cysts—some gelatinous, some caseous, some poorly calcified. There were hair follicles, nerve tissue, cartilage and fat within the tumour. In addition numerous teeth were developing. There was no evidence of malignancy, and the right ovary was normal.

Non-Mineralized Neoplasms

Fibro-Ameloblastoma

Fibro-ameloblastoma is an uncommon neoplasm appearing generally in the molar region of the mandible of young patients (Figure 333). These slow-growing tumours have a large connective tissue content with scat-

Figure 333. *Intra-oral radiograph of a fibro-ameloblastoma of a girl aged 11 years. There is a 'solid' appearance to this honeycombed lesion above and in front of unerupted ⎣7. The tooth has been displaced downwards and backwards by the tumour, and the crypt appears to be involved.*

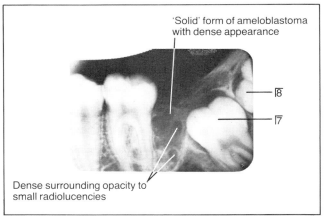

'Solid' form of ameloblastoma with dense appearance

⎣8

⎣7

Dense surrounding opacity to small radiolucencies

tered cords and rests of epithelial cells. They have been known to present a unilocular outline but a radiolucent honeycombed appearance is more usual.

Malignant Epithelial Neoplasms

Odontogenic Neoplasms

Epithelioma from Dental Remnants

This is a very rare form of neoplasm indeed.

Non-Odontogenic Neoplasms

Carcinoma

Epidermoid carcinoma is the most common of the malignant epithelial neoplasms, with involvement of bone generally a late feature. In the jaws, erosion of the bony surface is followed by invasion of the cortex, the radiographic appearance being a radiolucent spreading destruction with ill-defined borders.

Carcinoma of the floor of the mouth results in early extension into the lingual mucosa and lingual plate of mandibular bone. Carcinoma of the gingiva tends to arise in edentulous areas and soon involves the alveolar bone. Figure 334a shows a carcinoma of the edentulous mandible in the 6-3⌐ region. There has been destruction of the upper border and invasion of the medullary bone as far as the lower border. The scalloped margin of bone destruction is well shown. A more invasive appearance is evident in Figure 334b in ⌐6 region. The patient refused to have any treatment at this stage and disappeared for six weeks. On her return, the lesion had grown considerably, there was a pathological fracture of the body of the mandible in ⌐6 region and the growth had extended forwards and destroyed the bone surrounding ⌐5. The unusual feature in this case is that the

Figure 334 (a). *Part of a Panorex radiograph showing carcinoma of an edentulous mandible in 6-3⌐ region, with destruction of the upper border and infiltration of the bone to the lower border. The typical scalloped margin of the destruction is evident.* (b) *Part of a Panelipse radiograph of a woman aged 26 years. There is extensive destruction of the alveolus and body of the left mandible and the irregular invasive border is readily evident. The patient refused treatment at the time of this radiograph, but returned six weeks later, with a pathological fracture due to erosion of the lower border, and by then ⌐5 had lost all bony support.* (c) *True occlusal view of the mandible of a man aged 89 years with carcinoma spreading across the midline and showing marked bone destruction. The invasive nature of the lesion is very apparent, and the pathology report stated, 'Well differentiated squamous cell carcinoma with mononuclear cell infiltration'.* (d) *Part of a Panorex radiograph of a woman aged 60 years showing extensive carcinoma of the right angle of the mandible. There is a marked scalloped margin to the lesion, and 6⌐ is devoid of bony support. There is the suggestion of maxillary involvement in the tuberosity region, on this film, but better views are required to confirm this. The patient suffers from gross periodontal disease.*

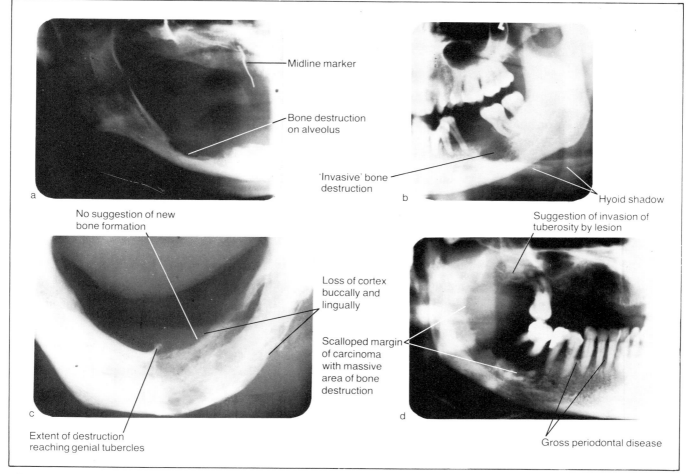

a — Midline marker
— Bone destruction on alveolus

b — 'Invasive' bone destruction
— Hyoid shadow

No suggestion of new bone formation

Loss of cortex buccally and lingually

Scalloped margin of carcinoma with massive area of bone destruction

c — Extent of destruction reaching genial tubercles

d — Suggestion of invasion of tuberosity by lesion
— Gross periodontal disease

patient was only 26 years of age. Figure 334c, a true lower occlusal radiograph, demonstrates carcinoma of the mandible in a man aged 89 years, crossing the midline, and showing a large radiolucent area of bone destruction. Buccal and lingual plates have been eroded, but the depth of the lesion cannot be assessed from this radiograph. The pathology report confirmed the diagnosis as squamous cell carcinoma.

Figure 334d shows an extensive carcinoma of the angle of the right mandible in a woman aged 60 years. The margin of bone destruction is depicted by a markedly scalloped outline, and there is the suggestion that

Figure 335 (a). *Oblique lateral and posteroanterior views of a man aged 63 years, showing radiolucent metastases in the skull vault and right mandible, from a carcinoma of the bronchus. The skull view was taken six weeks after the oblique lateral. The lesions show destruction of the buccal and lingual mandibular cortices. There is no suggestion of new bone formation.* **(b)** *Posteroanterior and oblique lateral views of a woman aged 44 years showing the radiolucent appearance of bone destruction in the $\overline{}8$ region and at the angle of the mandible due to a metastosis from the breast. Destruction of some buccal cortex is evident and the bone has a mottled appearance. There is no suggestion of new bone formation.* **(c)** *Lower occlusal radiographs of a man with a sclerosing metastasis from the prostate. The original outline of the mandible can still be seen though there has been considerable new bone formation. The condition was controlled with stilboestrol.*

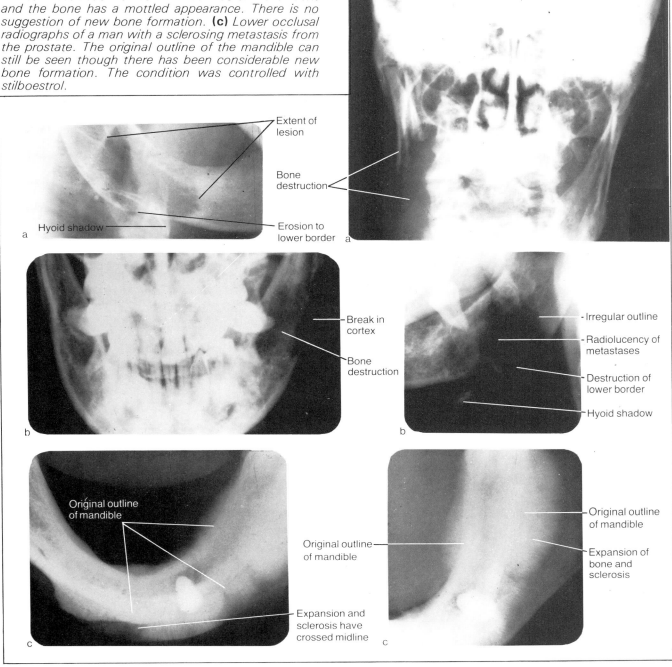

the maxillary tuberosity is also involved in the lesion. Intra-oral and occipitomental radiographs should confirm or refute this finding. 6| has lost all bone support and has been displaced by the extending growth. Carcinoma of the maxillary antrum may arise from the antral lining mucosa or by extension from the oral mucosa of the maxilla. Whilst early diagnosis of the former is very difficult as it is hidden from clinical examination, there is a likelihood of the latter appearing visually at an early stage, and being treated successfully. Early radiographic appearances of carcinoma of the antrum, from within, may only present as mucosal thickening or slight erosion of the antral walls, and may be hard to differentiate from sinusitis. The possibility of malignancy should always be considered.

Metastases

Metastases from primary carcinoma of such sites as the bronchus, breast, kidney and prostate may be found in the marrow space of the mandible, mainly in the molar region of the body and the ramus. The lesions may be well-delineated, or irregular, in outline. Figure 335a demonstrates radiolucent metastases in the skull vault and right mandible from a primary carcinoma of the bronchus of a man aged 63 years. There has been both buccal and lingual destruction of the cortex in the mandible, and there is no suggestion of new bone formation in this radiolucent lesion. The invasive nature characteristic of a primary carcinoma is not evident.

A secondary lesion from a carcinoma of the breast is shown in Figure 335b. The radiographs of this 44-year-old woman show radiolucent destruction of bone in the |8 region, and at the angle of the left mandible involving the buccal cortex, but there is no suggestion of new bone formation.

Carcinoma of the prostate has metastasized to the jaw

in Figure 335c. The lower occlusal radiographs show an extensive area of bone sclerosis with a sunray appearance radiating out from the molar region of the left mandible. The original bony contour of the mandible is still evident through the opacity of the new bone formed, both subperiosteally and within the tumour. The patient was treated with stilboestrol which controlled the tumour growth.

Melanoma

Melanoma is an uncommon malignant tumour of the oral mucosa appearing mainly on the maxillary alveolar ridge and palate. There may be little or no radiological evidence to support its clinical presence (Figure 336 and Plate 4). In this example there is the suggestion of minimal erosion of the left side of the floor of the nasal fossa above the apex of |1 on the radiograph, though the clinical picture suggests a pigmented lesion of considerable size. The lesion was excised but metastases presented in the cervical lymph glands within a year.

Adenocarcinoma

Adenocarcinoma of the jaws is rare, and radiographic appearances are similar to that of squamous cell carcinoma. Figure 337 illustrates adenocarcinoma of the right maxillary antrum with an obvious malignant destructive appearance. However, the diagnosis could only be made after histological investigation.

Figure 337. *Occipitomental view of a woman aged 63 years with an adenocarcinoma of the right antrum. The bony margins of the antrum have been destroyed. In addition there is marked mucosal thickening of the left antrum. Metastases were found later in the right angle of the jaws and in the lungs.*

Figure 336. *Radiograph of a woman aged 31 years with a malignant melanoma of the maxilla. There are minimal radiographic changes evident, but slight erosion of the floor of the nasal fossa can be seen over the apex of |1. The lesion was excised, but metastases presented in the cervical lymph glands one year later.*

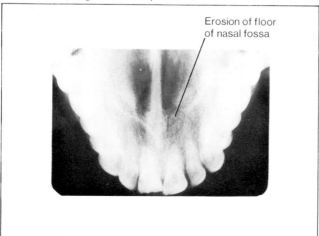

Erosion of floor of nasal fossa

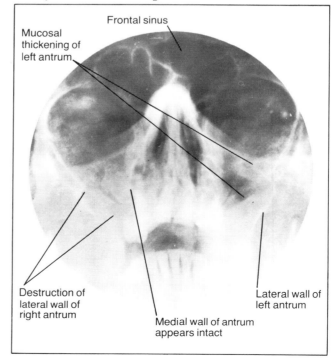

Frontal sinus

Mucosal thickening of left antrum

Destruction of lateral wall of right antrum

Medial wall of antrum appears intact

Lateral wall of left antrum

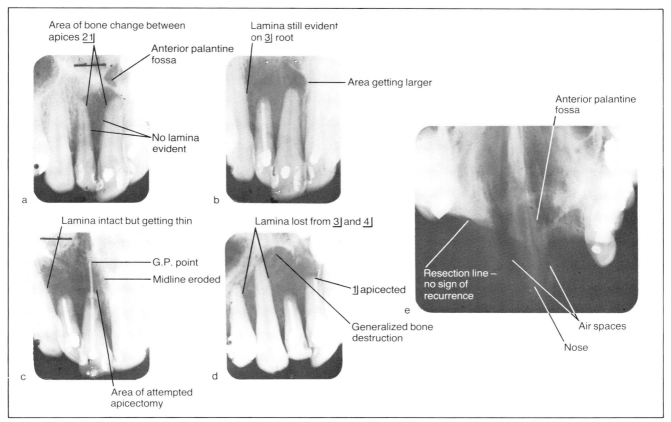

Figure 338. *Intra-oral radiographs of a man aged 34 years at presentation extending over a period of nearly four years.* **(a)** *Area of bone change is evident at the apices and between the roots of 21̲| with absence of lamina. The border of this radiolucent area is irregular and there is the suggestion that it reaches 3̲| region at the septal crest between 32̲|.* **(b)** *Three months later 2̲| had been root filled, apicectomied, and the area cleaned out over the apex. The area of radiolucency appears more extensive and with a rather vague border. It has reached the midline and involves the apex of 1̲|.* **(c)** *Two months later 1̲| has been root filled and there is the impression of a groove across the root suggesting attempted apicectomy. The root canal filling GP point extends well up through the apex, and the radiolucent area of bone destruction appears larger with a thinned lamina mesially on 3̲|.* **(d)** *Apicectomy has been performed on 1̲|, but the area of bone change has now reached 4̲|, and 43̲| have both lost their supporting lamina. At this stage a biopsy showed the area to contain a fibrosarcoma.* **(e)** *Three years after resection and radiotherapy the occlusal radiograph shows no evident of recurrence.*

Figure 339. *Radiological appearance of a chondro-sarcoma of the left maxilla of a woman aged 34 years. There is an irregular radiolucent area of bone destruction between and above |34̲, and |4̲ has been displaced distally. The lamina is absent and there is possibly some slight erosion of |4̲ roots. Hemi-resection of the maxilla was performed.*

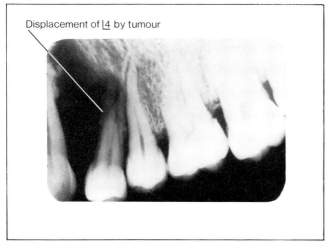

Displacement of |4̲ by tumour

Malignant Mesothelial Neoplasms

Osteogenic Neoplasms

Fibrosarcoma, Chondrosarcoma and Osteosarcoma

Sarcomas appear in the relatively young patient and few metastasize.

According to Stafne (1958) the periosteum and maxillary antrum are favourite sites for fibrosarcoma. Early bone changes are evident (unlike carcinoma) and there may be no demarcation with the surrounding normal bone. Figure 338a, b, c and d, illustrates stages through the treatment of a periapical area between the apices of 21̲| in a man aged 34 years over a period of six months. The initial appearance was certainly one of periapical bone change and led to an extended course of treatment to both 2̲| and 1̲|. The lack of response to treatment finally aroused suspicions of neoplasia, so a biopsy was taken, and the pathology report showed fibrosarcoma. Resection of the anterior aspect of the maxilla was performed, followed by radiotherapy to the region, and on a follow-up standard occlusal radiograph three years later (Figure 338e) there was no sign of any recurrence.

Chondrosarcoma may arise in the maxilla or mandible, the area sometimes appearing opaque due to calcification of the neoplastic cartilage. The bone is usually expanded and there is generally a rather irregular outline to the lesion. Figure 339 shows the radiographic appearance of a chondrosarcoma of the left maxilla in a woman aged 34 years. The radiolucent area of bone destruction is quite clear on the radiograph. $\lfloor 4$ has been displaced distally and the lamina is missing. The radiolucency above and between $\lfloor 34$, points to

Figure 340. *Periapical and occlusal radiographic views of a man aged 32 years with a large swelling in $\overline{\lceil 6}$ region. With only periapical views available $\overline{\lceil 6}$ was suspected as being abscessed and was removed. There was no pus. $\overline{\lceil 5}$ and 8 have bone destruction at the apices and the bone from $\overline{\lceil 5-8}$ region is very sclerotic in appearance. The occlusal view taken after extraction of $\overline{\lceil 6}$ shows large areas of bone formation buccally and lingually, much of which is periosteal bone, but some of which is tumour bone. This is an osteogenic sarcoma.*

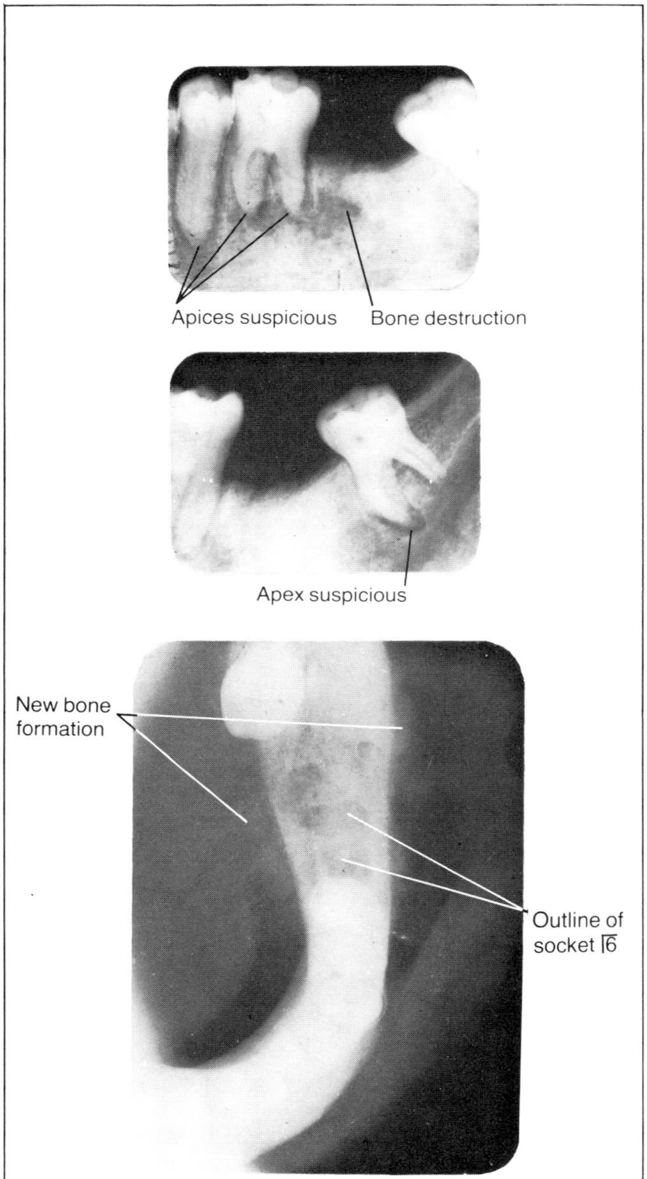

Apices suspicious   Bone destruction

Apex suspicious

New bone formation

Outline of socket $\overline{\lceil 6}$

bone destruction, and to no calcification within the tumour mass.

Osteosarcoma may present radiographically as areas of osteosclerosis or osteolysis. In the former there is excessive bone production (Figure 340), sometimes creating a sunray appearance. In the latter there is an irregular radiolucent area of bone destruction leading to expansion and destruction of the cortical plate, sometimes followed by pathological fracture. There is often a previous history of trauma before sarcoma presents.

Non-Osteogenic Neoplasms

Malignant Neurofibroma, Myosarcoma and Liposarcoma

The presence of these rare tumours is seldom reported in

Figure 341. *Posteroanterior and oblique lateral views of a woman aged 30 years, with a liposarcoma of the left ramus, angle and third molar region. There is buccal expansion and thinning of the cortex, leaving a bumpy outline. The lesion is made up of radiolucent cyst-like cavities surrounded by incomplete trabeculations. Excision of the left mandible was performed and a bone graft inserted. This was lost later due to suppuration.*

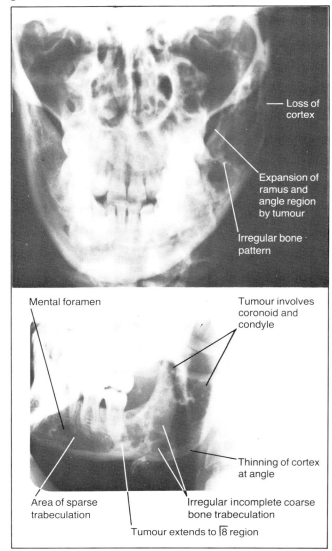

Loss of cortex

Expansion of ramus and angle region by tumour

Irregular bone pattern

Mental foramen

Tumour involves coronoid and condyle

Thinning of cortex at angle

Area of sparse trabeculation

Irregular incomplete coarse bone trabeculation

Tumour extends to $\overline{\lceil 8}$ region

the jaws. Liposarcoma of the left ramus, angle and third molar region is shown in Figure 341. The lesion appears to be made up of multiple cyst-like cavities surrounded by incomplete trabeculations. The patient, a woman aged 30 years, had hemi-resection of the mandible and a bone graft inserted. Unfortunately, the latter sloughed away due to suppuration after some weeks, but the patient managed very well without it.

Figure 342. *Myelomatous deposits in the skull vault. Many varying sized punched-out radiolucent areas are evident, and destruction of the cortex can be seen in several places. There is no evidence of new bone formation.*

Myeloma

This condition arises in the bone marrow, sometimes as a single, but more often as a multiple lesion. The cortex becomes involved only by extension of the lesion. The primary lesion may arise in the jaws, when radiographically the appearance is of multiple punched-out circular regions of radiolucency which are sometimes diffuse. There does not appear to be any bony reaction to the lesions, and there is little evidence of cortical expansion. Skull radiographs clearly show the multiple lesions (Figure 342), the usual sites in the jaws being the angle and molar regions of the mandible, where pathological fractures may occur.

Conclusion

It has not been possible to cover all the neoplasms that can present in the jaws, but the reader will have gathered that a wide variety of appearances can present on radiographs when viewing neoplasia. It is worth repeating that the possibility of neoplasia should be considered when examining 'vague appearances' on radiographs, and if in doubt it is better to refer a patient with suspected neoplasia than to await further developments.

References

Stafne, E. C., *Oral Roentgenographic Diagnosis.* W. B. Saunders Co., Philadelphia, USA, 1958.

Worth, H. M.,*Principles and Practice of Oral Radiologic Interpretation.* Year Book Medical Publishers Inc, Chicago, 1963.

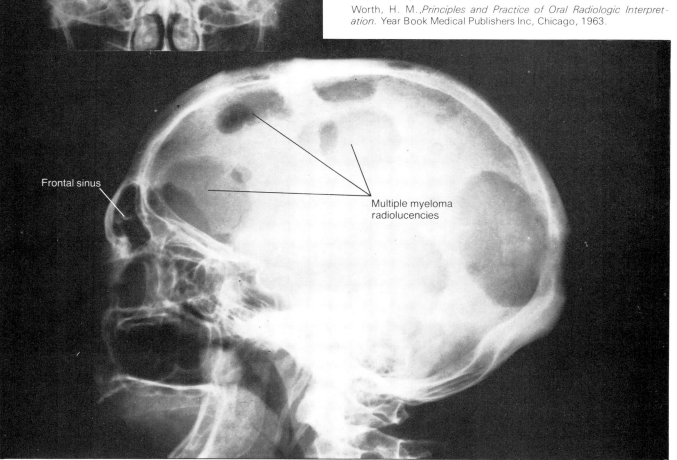

9. Osteodystrophies Involving the Skull and Jaws

Fibrous Dysplasia

The aetiology of fibrous dysplasia is unknown. It is a benign disease arising between infancy and early adulthood characterised by resorption of normal bone and its replacement by poorly formed new bone and fibrous tissue. Females are more often affected than males. The bone growth may be considerable, but it is usually slow, and the process generally stops when skeletal growth is complete. Sometimes the involved area continues to enlarge slowly after normal growth has ceased.

Bone and fibrous tissue may be laid down in very variable quantities in different lesions, hence radiographic appearances of fibrous dysplasia can be quite different from one case to another.

It is common practice nowadays to include ossifying fibroma and fibro-osteoma, together with Albright's syndrome and Cherubism, as variants of fibrous dysplasia, though the correctness of this grouping has not been settled for certain.

The disease can present in monostotic or polyostotic forms, and it is convenient to discuss the radiographic appearances under these two headings.

Monostotic Fibrous Dysplasia

Only one bone is involved in this lesion and Figure 343 illustrates subclinical monostotic fibrous dysplasia of 6⌋ region in a woman aged 37 years. There is slight thickening of the alveolar process in 65⌋ region. Just posterior to 5⌋ there is very dense opaque bone and this is surrounded by a fine patterned bone which merges into normal bone beyond.

Much larger lesions may be found in the maxilla, and these will often expand to take up the antral space and thicken the antral wall and infraorbital margin (Figure 344). The occipitomental view suggests a very radio-opaque lesion because of the marked thickening. The occlusal radiograph of the same patient, aged 14 years,

Figure 343. *Intra-oral radiographs of a woman aged 37 years with a subclinical lesion of fibrous dysplasia posterior to 5⌋. There is slight thickening of the alveolar process in this region which was not evident on the patient's face. An area of dense opaque bone is just posterior to 5⌋ root, and this area is surrounded by a region of fine-patterned bone which merges into normal bone.*

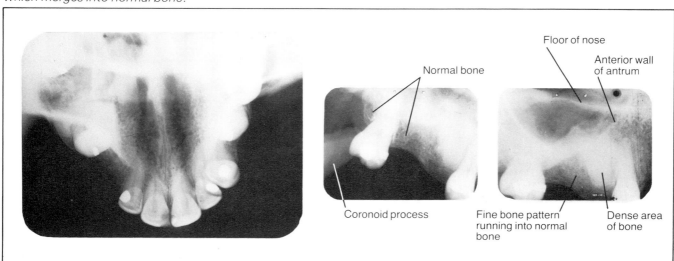

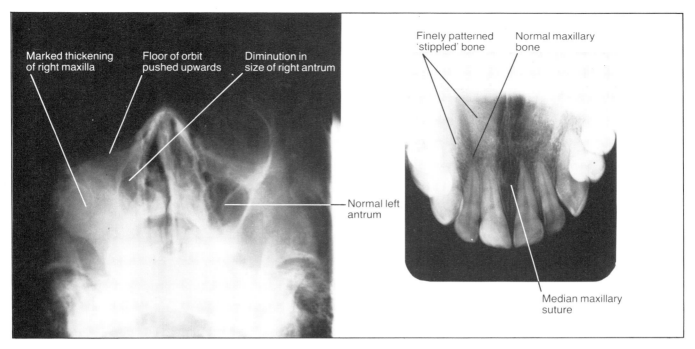

Figure 344. *Occipitomental and standard occlusal views of a boy aged 14 years with fibrous dysplasia of the right maxilla. There is fine-patterned bone, appearing dense because of the marked thickening, replacing normal cancellous bone over the right premolars and molars. The right lateral antral wall is grossly thickened inwards and outwards, and the right inferior orbital margin is similarly affected. The stippled bone on the occlusal radiograph merges into normal bone in 21| region.*

shows detail of the stippled orange-peel appearance that is so often characteristic of the lesion of fibrous dysplasia. The stippled bone merges into normal bone in 21| region.

A different pattern exhibited by the bone in fibrous dysplasia is seen in the intraoral radiographs of a woman aged 37 years (Figure 345). Anterior to the dense opaque bone in the region of the tuberosity are fine bone patterns reminiscent of fingerprints. Within these fingerprint areas are zones of radiolucency which suggest a higher concentration of fibrous tissue. There is an isolated island of dense bone just distal to the canine root. The abnormal bone pattern merges into normal bone in the canine region.

Fibrous dysplasia appears more frequently in the maxilla than in the mandible, but may present with

Figure 345. *Intra-oral radiographic views of a woman aged 37 years with fibrous dysplasia of the right maxillary alveolus. Finger-print whorls of altered bone can be seen anterior to the dense bone in the tuberosity. An isolated patch of dense bone is evident just distal to 3|, and mesial to this tooth the bone pattern is normal.*

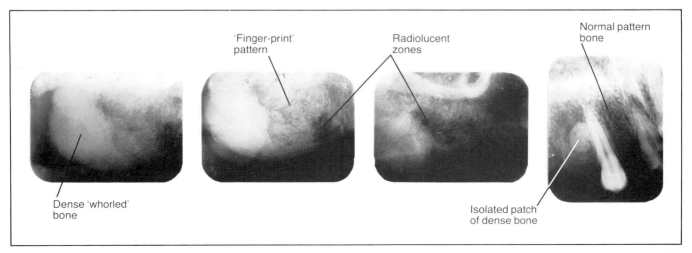

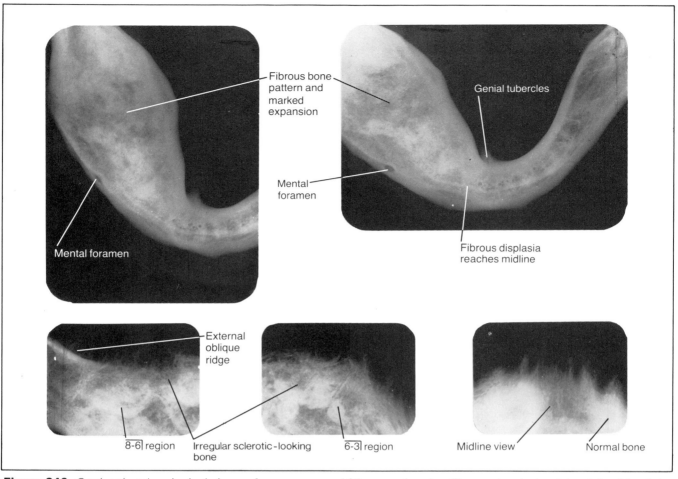

Fibrous bone pattern and marked expansion

Genial tubercles

Mental foramen

Mental foramen

Fibrous displasia reaches midline

External oblique ridge

8-6 region

Irregular sclerotic-looking bone

6-3 region

Midline view

Normal bone

Figure 346. *Occlusal and periapical views of a woman aged 31 years showing fibrous dysplasia of the right side of the mandible. There is marked swelling, mainly lingually, and the altered 'smoky-patterned' bone extends as far as the midline. Follow-up radiographs (not shown) indicate no change in the size of the lesion over a period of 8 years. The growth itself took place during the formative years.*

marked swelling of the latter (Figure 346). The patient, a woman aged 31, had a long-standing enlargement of the right side of the mandible, mainly lingually and downwards, from 8̄| region to the symphysis. An irregular smokey-patterned bone shows areas of sclerosis and radiolucency, and the mental foramen can be seen as an oval radiolucency near the buccal border in 5̄4̄| region. A biopsy report advised 'fibrous dysplasia'. The lesion appeared to have remained static in follow-up radiographs over a period of 8 years.

Polyostotic Fibrous Dysplasia

Several bones are involved in this form of fibrous dysplasia, the condition is usually unilateral, and the radiographic appearances of the lesions may be the same as the monostotic variety.

Marked bone density changes may be evident in fibrous dysplasia, and Figure 347 demonstrates a dense ground-glass appearance of the left maxilla and left mandible on the intraoral radiographs of this woman aged 23 years.

In the maxilla a number of deciduous teeth have been retained and there has been little physiological root resorption. The unerupted permanent teeth involved in the bone change have fully developed roots (root resorption is sometimes a feature of fibrous dysplasia). Although the bone changes reach the midline, and may have prevented |1 from erupting fully, they do not appear to have crossed the median maxillary suture. There was some thickening evident clinically from |C-5 region.

In the mandible the region of altered bone almost reaches the midline, and again there are unerupted teeth with fully formed roots evident, with the mandibular canal running across the apices. An interesting feature is the possible persistence of the gubernaculum to |345 which can be seen as a radiolucent tract running up from the crypt of each of these teeth towards the upper border of the alveolus. The right side of the jaws is normal.

Although fibrous dysplasia is a benign disease there have been reports of sarcomatous changes (Tanner et al. 1961).

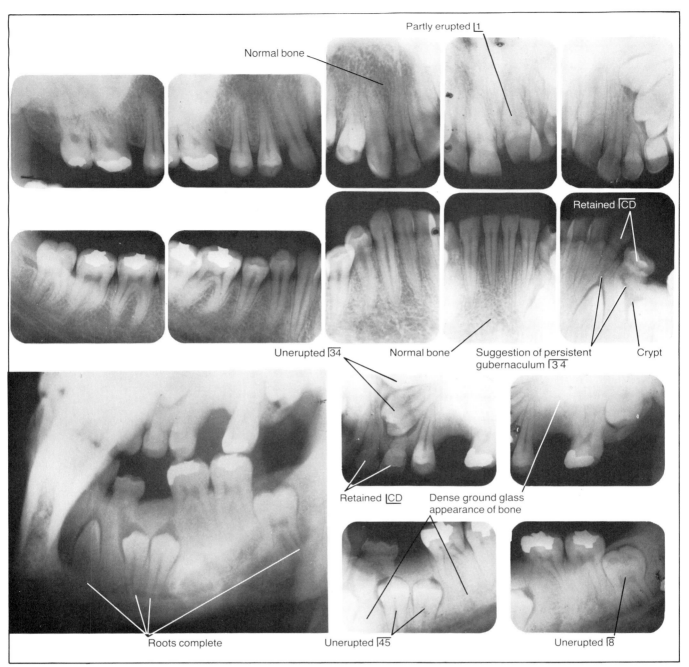

Figure 347. *Full-mouth periapical and left oblique lateral views of a woman aged 23 years with polyostotic fibrous dysplasia of the left <u>maxilla</u> and left side of the mandible. $\frac{CD}{CD}$ are still present; $\frac{348}{3458}$ are unerupted; $\underline{|1}$ is partly erupted, and $\underline{|6}$ is absent. $\overline{|3458}$ are low down in the mandible, vertically placed and with complete roots. There is the suggestion of persistence of the gubernaculum from $\overline{|345}$, evident as radiolucent bands reaching upwards from the apices of the crypts. The bone is very opaque in the alveolus of the left side of the jaws, giving a ground-glass appearance, and merges into normal bone near the midline.*

There are no changes in the serum calcium and alkaline phosphatase levels.

Albright's Syndrome

In addition to many bones showing the changes of fibrous dysplasia in this very rare syndrome, there is skin pigmentation and hypergonadism.

Figure 348 shows the radiographic views of a boy with gross thickening of the frontal bone, skull base and maxilla, producing the appearance of leontiasis ossea. The cortices of these bones are very thinned and the bones themselves show a fine even pattern. Several bones other than the skull showed changes of fibrous dysplasia, and the patient had suffered recurrent fractures of a femur. He also had café-au-lait patches on

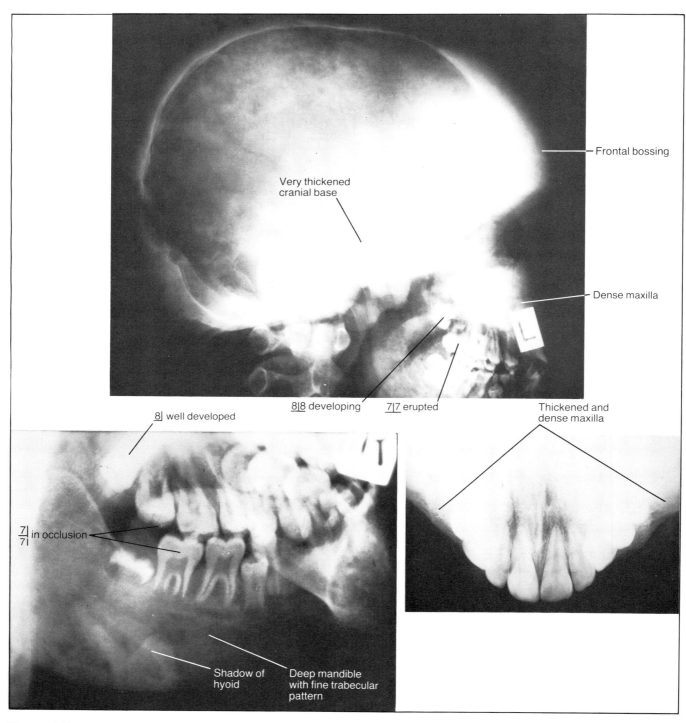

Figure 348. *Lateral skull, oblique lateral and occlusal views of a boy aged 9 years with Albright's syndrome. There is marked thickening of the skull base, frontal bone and maxilla, producing the appearance of Leontiasis Ossea. The bones themselves show a fine even pattern. A great increase in vertical height of the mandible can be seen, and it is also evident that $\frac{7|}{7|}$ are in occlusion. The latter is an indication of the precocious sexual development of the patient. His voice was breaking too!*

the skin. From the oblique lateral view it can be seen that the vertical height of the mandible is greatly increased. The second permanent molars are in occlusion in this boy aged 9 years, which is evidence of hypergonadism, and at this very early stage his voice was breaking. In Albright's syndrome it is usual for hypergonadism to appear in females rather than males.

Cherubism

This is a rare, sometimes familial, form of fibrous dysplasia which is quite specific in distribution. Marked symmetrical expansion of the mandible near the angle, and sometimes the maxilla in the molar regions, occurs, and the radiographic appearance is of radiolucent cyst-like areas with an outline cortex of irregular thickness.

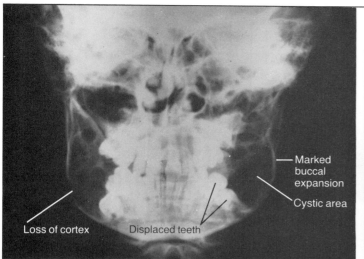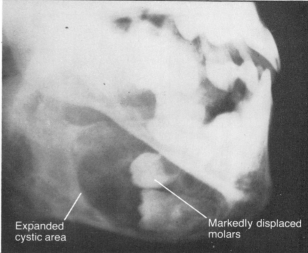

Figure 349. *Radiographic views of a boy aged 8 years with familial fibrous dysplasia, or Cherubism. Marked buccal swellings of the mandible are evident in the posteroanterior radiograph, with destruction of the cortex on the right side. There is evidence of trabeculation within the cyst-like radiolucencies.* $\overline{6|}$ *appears to have been displaced to the lower border, and a number of unerupted and forming teeth can be seen within the radiolucent areas. The maxilla is also involved, and the result of the swellings can be seen in Plate 5.*

Trabeculations are usually evident and these may be irregular in form.

Figure 349 illustrates such a case, and unerupted teeth can be seen deep in the radiolucent areas of the mandible. There is marked buccal expansion and thinning of the cortex—particularly on the right side.

The maxilla is also involved on both sides, and the generalised swelling results in the wide face and puffy appearance seen in Plate 5. This boy, aged 8 years, does not show the characteristic 'eyes-heavenwards' expression of cherubism where the lower eyelids are pulled downwards by gross swelling of the cheeks to expose the white sclera.

Paget's Disease

The aetiology of this disease is unknown but it generally occurs in the elderly. Unlike fibrous dysplasia when considering the jaws, the whole of the bone concerned shows changes. The cranial vault and maxilla are more often affected than the mandible.

First Stage

Osteoporosis is the first stage and is seen on the radiograph as a thinning of the trabeculae and lamina dura. Figure 350a shows this appearance in the mandible of a woman aged 68 years, with many fine trabeculations running in the direction of the length of the bone in the molar region. Further anteriorly the trabeculations appear to run in a vertical direction. The lamina dura is very thin.

In the lateral skull view of the same patient (Figure 350b) the characteristic appearance of osteoporosis cir-

cumscripta can be seen outlining the posterior extent of the porosis of the frontal bone. Thinning of the cortex is also evident in the anterior aspect of the skull vault.

Figure 350c, a lateral skull view of the same patient taken 10 years later, shows how the porosis has progressed across the skull reaching as far back as the occipital bone.

Second Stage

In Figure 350a the second stage of Paget's disease can be seen in the maxilla. Enlargement is taking place and dense sclerotic bone can be seen in the tooth bearing part of the alveolus. No lamina dura is evident, and it is hard to say whether it is hypercementosis or sclerotic bone surrounding the apex of $\underline{|5}$ root. $\overline{3|}$ does show some hypercementosis at the apex. It is important to notice that the sclerotic appearance is evident across the whole of the maxilla, which helps in the differential diagnosis of fibrous dysplasia when the patient's age is also taken into account.

Teeth separate in the expanded maxilla, and periodontal membrane shadows are lost with the increased thickening. In the skull view (Figure 350c) both stages of the disease can be seen, with 'cotton-wool' patches developing in arrears of the advancing porosis, and thickening of the calvarium in the frontal and parietal regions taking place.

Late Stage

Figure 351 shows the late stage of Paget's disease in a woman aged 81 years. The edentulous mandible is normal.

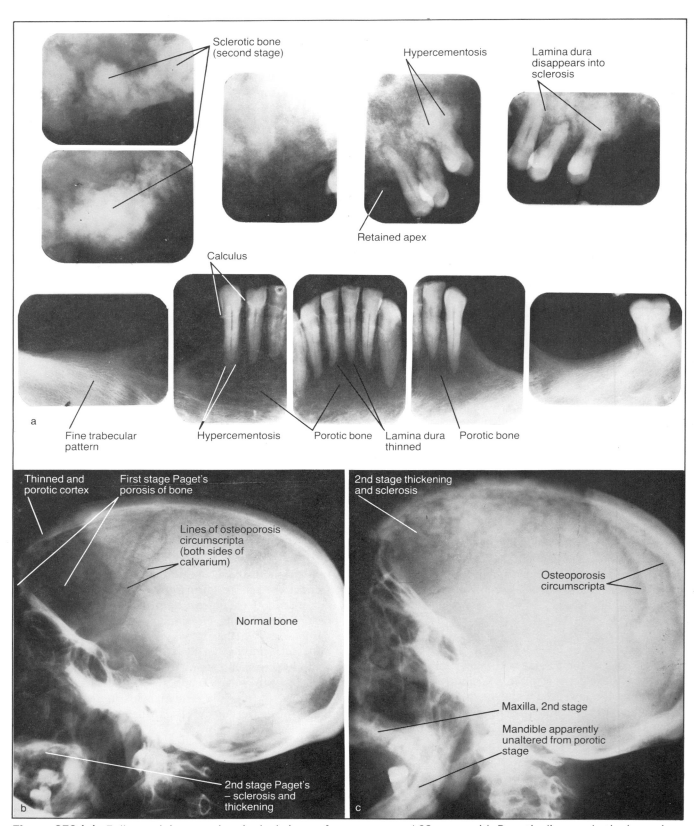

Figure 350 (a). *Full mouth intra-oral periapical views of a woman aged 68 years with Paget's disease. In the lower jaw the bone is very porotic with thin horizontal trabeculations in the molar region following the length of the bone. Anteriorly the trabeculations appear to run vertically. Lamina dura surrounding the teeth has thinned dramatically. In the maxilla the second stage of the disease is shown; cotton-wool patches and bone thickening have occurred. There is a dense opaque patch over ⌊5 root apex, and this is hard to differentiate from hypercementosis (which may occur at the same time). The bone outside the sclerotic area is very fine in appearance.* **(b)** *Lateral skull view of the same patient as (a) showing the characteristic appearance of osteoporosis circumscripta. Thinning of the skull cortex in the frontal region is evident.* **(c)** *Appearance 10 years after (b). The porosis has extended to the occipital bone, and the sclerotic patches of the second stage of Paget's disease are evident further forwards in the skull vault.*

138

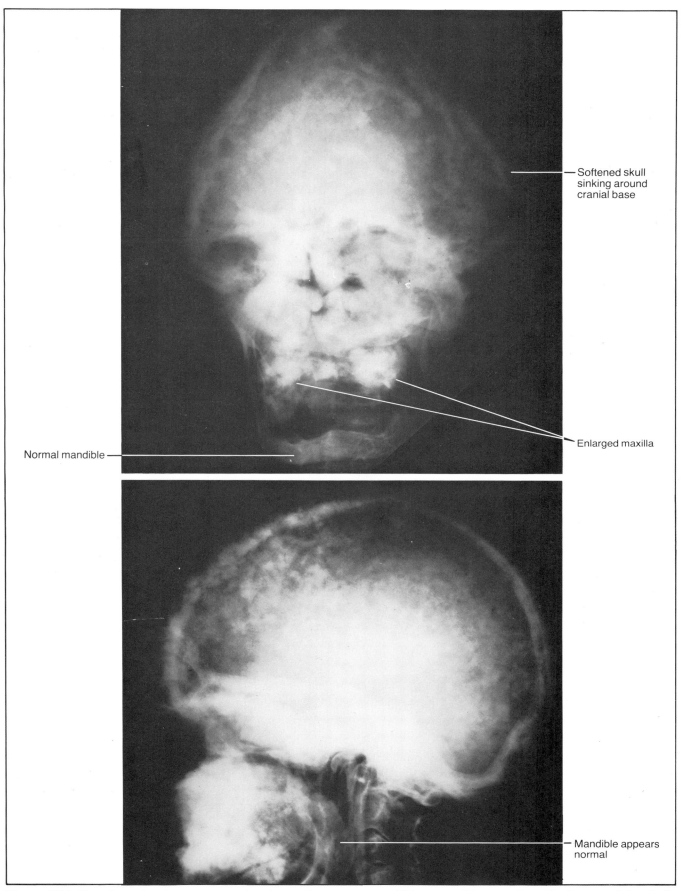

Softened skull
sinking around
cranial base

Enlarged maxilla

Normal mandible

Mandible appears
normal

Figure 351. *True lateral and posteroanterior views of a woman aged 81 years with gross Paget's disease of the skull. Softening of the bones has resulted in basilar impression, giving a 'tam 'o shanter' appearance, and marked swelling of the frontal bone and maxilla has produced leontiasis ossea.*

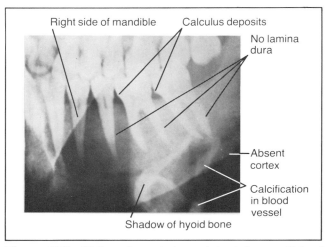

Right side of mandible   Calculus deposits

No lamina dura

Absent cortex

Calcification in blood vessel

Shadow of hyoid bone

Figure 352. *Oblique lateral view of the left mandible of a man aged 31 years with renal osteodystrophy, showing marked porosis. There is no cortex to the lower border and no suggestion of lamina dura surrounding the roots of the teeth. There is calculus round all the teeth and evidence of arterial calcification near the shadow of the hyoid bone.*

The altered bone of the skull is soft and this has resulted in basilar impression. Gross enlargement of the facial bones has produced the characteristic appearance of leontiasis ossea.

Infection with sequestration, pathological fracture and sarcomatous change can all occur in Paget's disease, but the last of these three conditions is very rare. Calcium levels are unaffected.

Hyperparathyroidism

Hyperparathyroidism is caused in two different ways:

1. Primary hyperparathyroidism arises from over-secretion of parathyroid hormone as a result of hyperplasia or adenoma of the parathyroid glands. The condition is generally seen in patients of middle age. Serum calcium levels are markedly raised, and the kidneys excrete calcium. To keep levels balanced calcium is removed from the bones by osteoclastic activity.

2. Secondary hyperparathyroidism arises as the result

Figure 353. *Lateral skull view of the same patient as Figure 352 showing the 'pepper-pot' skull resulting from extensive hyperparathyroidism.*

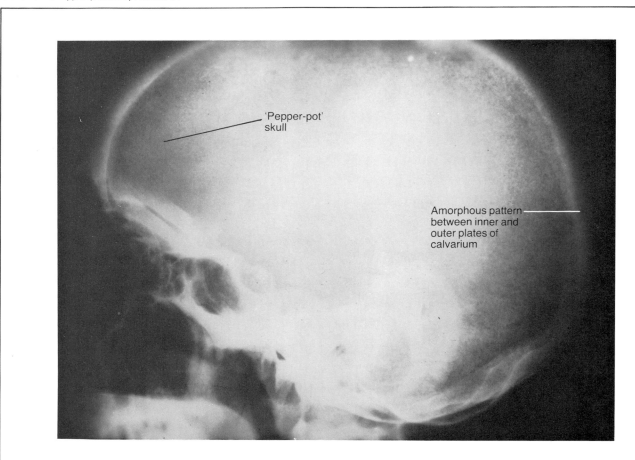

'Pepper-pot' skull

Amorphous pattern between inner and outer plates of calvarium

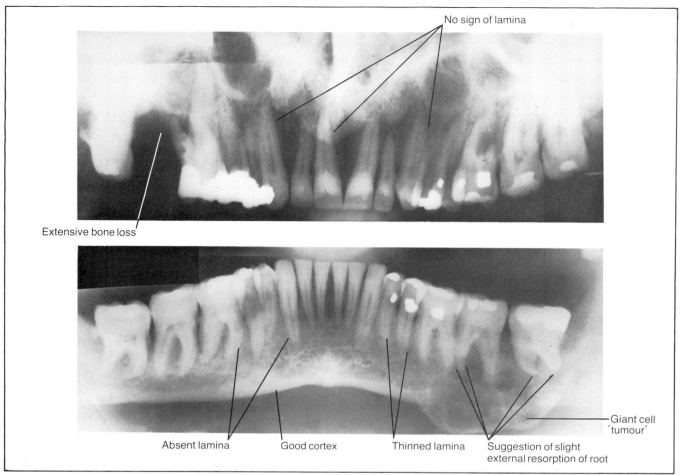

Figure 354. *Upper and lower Panoral (static panoramic) views of a man aged 39 years with giant-cell 'tumour' of the mandible resulting from hyperparathyroidism. Expansion of the jaw is evident in ⌐78 region with loss of density of the lower border, and some evidence of trabeculation. Roots of ⌐78 appear to show some resorption. The bone pattern is generally rather fine and the lamina dura is missing.*

of chronic renal disease where there is a severe upset of calcium and phosphorus metabolism.

Radiographic Appearances

Bone changes are the same in both forms of the disease. There may be generalised porosis, with loss of lamina, cortex and trabeculation, giving the jaws a 'ground glass' appearance (Figure 352). Probably the most significant factor, when it occurs, is loss of the lamina dura, but it should be remembered that this also occurs locally in Paget's disease and fibrous dysplasia.

Radiographs of the skull may show a 'pepper-pot' appearance (Figure 353) as the medullary bone and inner and outer cortices lose their differential pattern.

Where there are areas of extensive osteoclastic activity giant-cell 'tumours' may arise, with expansion of the bone and a single or multi-cystic appearance. Figure 354 shows a giant-cell 'tumour', indistinguishable from a central giant-cell reparative granuloma, expanding below the lower border of the mandible lingually in ⌐78

region. Slight resorption is evident on the roots of these teeth.

Hyperparathyroidism should always be suspected when isolated giant-cell 'tumours' are found in patients over 30 years of age. In the case of primary hyperparathyroidism these lesions will cure spontaneously after removal of the adenoma, and the lamina dura will reform around the tooth roots.

Evidence of hyperparathyroidism can be seen in other bones of the body, and Figure 355a shows the hands of a patient with this disease and also rheumatoid arthritis. Figure 355b shows the hands of a normal individual.

Cleido-cranial Dysostosis

In this rare and unusual disease there is failure of bone growth characterised by: persistent fontanelles and wide sutures in the skull; failure of clavicles to develop fully; multiple unerupted teeth; spina bifida in some cases, and a number of other bone growth delays or errors of development.

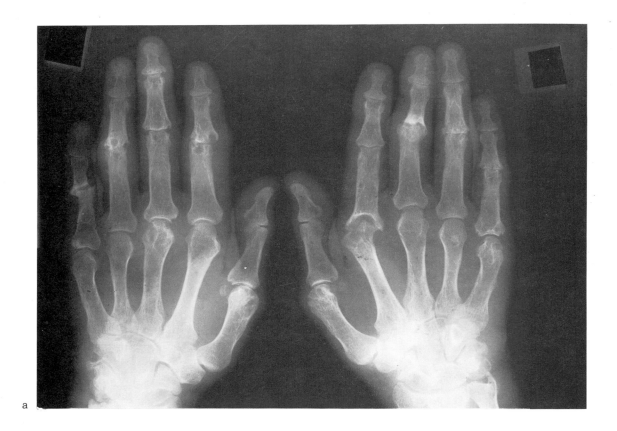

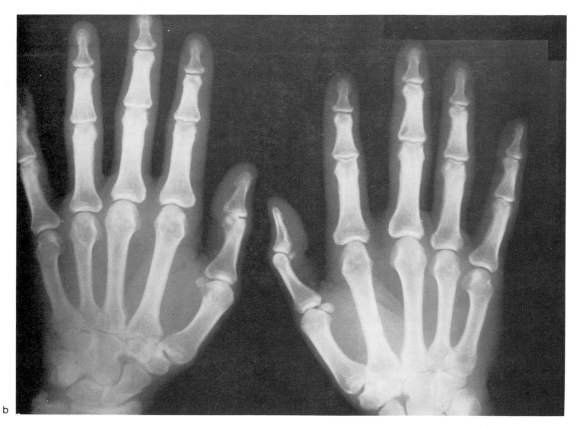

Figure 355 (a). *Radiographic views of the hands of the same patient as Figure 354 showing both rheumatoid arthritis and hyperparathyroidism changes.* **(b)** *Hands of normal individual for comparison with (a).*

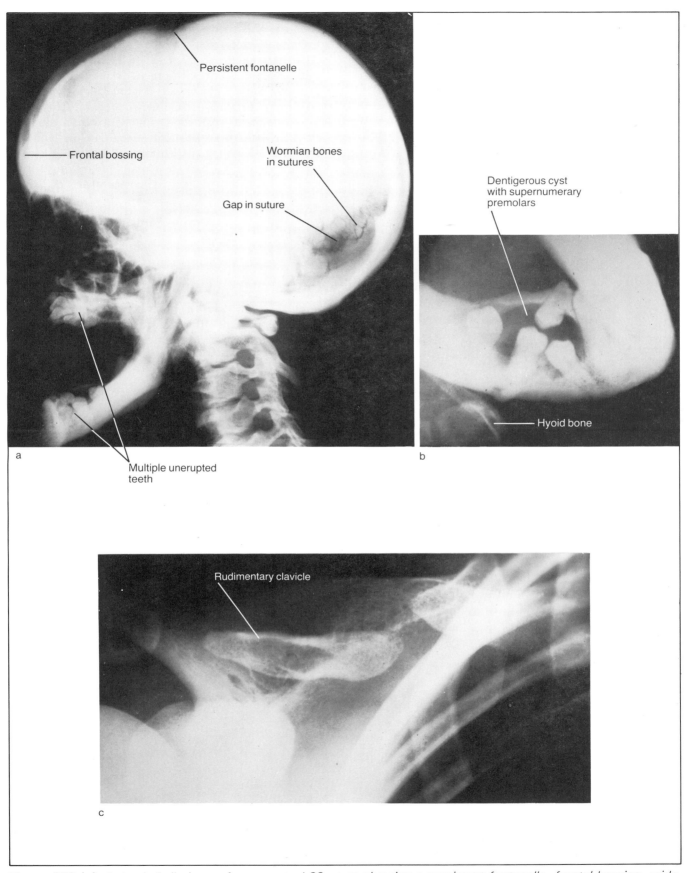

Figure 356 (a). *Lateral skull views of a man aged 38 years showing a persistent fontanelle, frontal bossing, wide sutures and wormian bones. In addition there are numerous unerupted teeth evident in both jaws.* **(b)** *Oblique lateral radiograph of the same patient as (a) showing markedly displaced unerupted supplemental premolars associated with a dentigerous cyst.* **(c)** *Radiographic view of the same patient as (a) and (b) showing a rudimentary right clavicle.*

A persistent fontanelle can be seen in the lateral skull view of a patient aged 38 years in Figure 356a. In addition small isolated bones with irregular outline, termed wormian bones, can be seen in the wide sutures, and the plates of bone are very thin. There is the suggestion of frontal bossing which is frequently associated with this condition.

Oblique lateral views of the mandible (Figure 356b) show unerupted and displaced supplemental premolar teeth of normal form with a related dentigerous cyst.

A view of the right clavicle (Figure 356c) shows this to be incomplete, and such a deficiency enables the patient to approximate the shoulders in the forward position—a characteristic feature of this disease (Plate 6).

Figure 357 is part of a radiograph of a child aged 18 months showing a persistent mandibular suture, rudimentary clavicles, and incomplete neural arches.

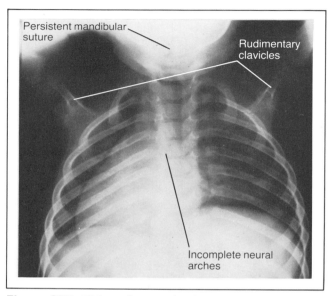

Figure 357. *This radiographic view of a child aged 18 months shows persistence of the median mandibular suture at the symphysis, incomplete neural arches, and rudimentary clavicles.*

Craniostenosis

Craniostenosis is a rare condition caused by early ossification of the skull suture lines. As a result normal growth of the skull vault is unable to take place, and pressure from the convolutions of the growing brain results in imprints of the inner plate giving it a 'copper-beaten' appearance (Figure 358). Fractures may occur and one can be seen in the right parietal region of this child aged 3 years.

Reference

Tanner, M. C., Daklin, D. C. and Childs, D. S., *Oral Surg., Oral Med., Oral Path.,* 1961, **14,** 837.

Figure 358. *True lateral and posteroanterior views of a 3 year-old child showing the 'copper-beaten' appearance of Craniostenosis caused by indentation of the inner plate of bone by the convolutions of the brain. The sutures have ossified early causing this condition. There is a fracture evident in the right parietal region.*

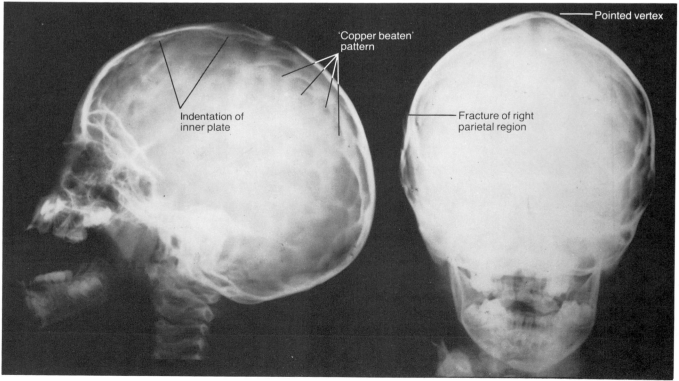

Index

Italic numerals refer to figure numbers.

147

Printed by Cradley Printing Co Ltd, Warley, West Midlands